Choosing a Nurse-Midwife

Your Guide to Safe, Sensitive Care During Pregnancy and the Birth of Your Child

Catherine M. Poole
Elizabeth A. Parr, CNM

To Valerie with best wishes Elizabeth A Parr.

John Wiley & Sons, Inc.
New York • Chichester • Brisbane • Toronto • Singapore

This book is dedicated to all women, everywhere. Our hope is that you find a health-care provider who will treat you with dignity and kindness, and who will also trust your intuition. We also dedicate this book to the midwives who frequently give up their night's sleep to provide this kind of care.

Copyright © 1994 by Catherine M. Poole and Elizabeth A. Parr, CNM
Published by John Wiley & Sons, Inc.

Library of Congress Cataloging-in-Publication Data
Poole, Catherine M., 1953–
    Choosing a nurse-midwife : your guide to safe, sensitive care
during pregnancy and the birth of your child / Catherine M. Poole
and Elizabeth A. Parr.
        p.   cm.
    Includes bibliographical references and index.
    ISBN 0-471-58452-5
    1. Midwives.   2. Prenatal care.   3. Childbirth.   I. Parr,
Elizabeth A., 1955– .   II. Title.
RG950.P66   1994
618.2'0233—dc20   93-33105

Printed in the United States of America

10   9   8   7   6   5   4   3   2   1

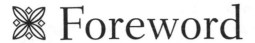 # Foreword

C*hoosing a Nurse-Midwife* is a wonderful, sensitive source that clearly addresses many of the questions consumers have regarding nurse-midwives. The authors describe the profession of nurse-midwifery, pointing out that it is once again assuming a growing role in the delivery of perinatal health services in this country. Provided are questions to ask the nurse-midwife before making a final decision about a provider, how to identify nurse-midwives in your own area, and how to determine when choosing a nurse-midwife is the right option for your family.

The book also describes the settings in which nurse-midwives practice, which range from urban hospitals to women's homes and include publicly supported clinics, health maintenance organizations, private practice groups, and birthing centers. The authors also place a strong emphasis on the quality and structure of services needed, given the underlying risks for each pregnancy. They stress that, like each child, every pregnancy is unique. The goal of service should be to provide individualized, accessible, culturally sensitive care that is responsive to the needs of families. For many families these needs will be best met by a nurse-midwife.

On an historical note, for nearly three centuries midwifery has been practiced in America. Perhaps the earliest account is found in Laura Thatcher Ulrich's Pulitzer Prize-winning book *A Midwife's Tale: The Life of Martha Ballard, Based on Her Diary, 1785–1812* (New York, Alfred A. Knopf, 1990). The author points out that whereas

> several doctors . . . occasionally attended births in Hallowell (Maine), their work was supplementary to that of the midwives. Martha herself attended 60 percent of the births (in 1878), and she was not the only female practitioner active at the time. Martha and her peers were not only handling most of the deliveries, they were providing much of the medical care as well. In Martha's diary, it is doctors, not midwives, who seem marginal. (P. 28)

Yet despite their long history, in the United States nurse-midwives were almost completely replaced by physicians during the twentieth century. Their gradual decline reflected several events, including the change to mostly hospital-based deliveries, poor access to training for nurse-midwives, and growing opposition by physicians. Fortunately, many of these factors are changing, as evidenced by the doubling of the number of births attended by nurse-midwives in the past decade to almost 150,000 in 1990. Also, due to the safe and highly satisfying care they provide, the popularity of nurse-midwives continues to rise rapidly. Nonetheless, recent surveys still identify large numbers of families who are not aware of nurse-midwives and the services they offer, underscoring the need for more information and resources to describe their role in perinatal health care.

Primarily due to consumer demand and health-care needs, the number of nurse-midwives in the United States is steadily growing, as is the number of women seeking their care. Today more than 4,500 certified nurse-midwives are practicing in all fifty states, with a projected goal of 10,000 CNMs by the year 2000. Women from all walks of life use midwifery services, including highly educated professionals, celebrities, and young teens, and they represent a socioeconomic spectrum from great affluence to those who are poverty stricken.

In the future, greater use of nurse-midwives will be crucial for solving many of the issues central to effective health-care reform. In this challenging climate, we must find ways to improve significantly birth outcomes through preventive services, including early and better risk assessment and preconceptional care. The nurse-midwife can be an integral part of this system.

The babies who die or who have birth defects keep reminding us of the work remaining to realize our vision for a world in which every baby is born healthy. With nurse-midwives assuming an increasing role as the specialists in normal birth, we can move closer to achieving this vision in the twenty-first century.

Jennifer L. Howse, Ph.D.
President, March of Dimes Birth Defects Foundation

Acknowledgments

We are grateful to the many Certified Nurse-Midwives who shared their professional stories and experiences as well as provided feedback about this book. These nurse-midwives include Catherine Carr, Joyce Daniel, Jennifer Dohrn, Pixie Elsberry, Kitty Ernst, Ann Gilmore, Martha Harvey, Richard Jennings, Karyn Kaufman, Karen Laing, Barbara Lee, Ruth Lubic, Marion McCartney, Sister Angela Murdaugh, Lisa Paine, Harriet Palmer, Marilinda Pascoe, Becky Skovgaard, Susan Stapleton, Lois Tresize, and Lisa Waldbaum. Also the story would not be complete without the personal stories shared with us by the many midwife clients and their partners. We are also grateful to Jane Brody, T. Berry Brazelton, Robbie Davis-Floyd, Don Creevy, Kate O'Hanlan, Sidney Wolf, and Jennifer Howse—all very busy people who gave us their time and valued opinions. Thanks also to the American College of Nurse-Midwives for its assistance.

To our agent, Jeanne Fredericks, we're appreciative of all her hard work on our behalf. We also thank our editor, Judith McCarthy, for her guidance on this project.

Catherine's Acknowledgments

I first would like to thank Carolyn Janik. She told me I should write a book about my midwife experience, and she remained a great friend during the effort. Thanks also to my editor from a previous life, David Bumke, who provided his usual on-target editorial advice. My friends Darlene Furey, Deborah Karably, Joan Ely, and Dave Clayton also kept me on track.

Thanks to my mother for scanning the *Washington Post* for me daily and my sisters for their support. To my children, Jesse and Carey, you instilled in me the desire to give you the best possible start in life that I could find, and you in turn gave up a lot of your time with me so I could let other women know how to have a wonderful birth too. I love you both very much. To my husband Bobby, my best friend and constant companion for the past 23 years, thank you for your love, patience, and support, and especially your help with the modem and computer! This book is personally dedicated to my father, who I think would be proud of me if he were here.

Elizabeth's Acknowledgments

I thank the following people who helped make this book possible: Marilinda Pascoe and Becky Skovgaard, CNMs, good friends who gave constant advice and support despite geographic distance.

Ruth Shiers, Katie Head, and other CNMs, staff, and clients of the Allentown–Bethlehem Birth and Midwifery Center, who taught me the art of midwifery.

My sisters Caroline, Louise, and Judy Parr, inveterate readers whose comments on the manuscript were always insightful.

Preston and Ruth Beardslee Parr, my parents, whose values led me to help women and whose faith in me and my work continues to encourage me.

And especially Ed Reibman, my husband, who never faltered in his support, from honest critiques of the text to caring for Sam while I wrote. He has enriched my work and my life.

❇ Contents

Introduction   *1*

PART I   Nurse-Midwives and Clients   *13*

    Chapter 1   Choosing a Nurse-Midwife   *15*

    Chapter 2   Can I Go to a Midwife?   *29*

PART II   Pregnancy, Labor, and Birth   *39*

    Chapter 3   Prenatal Care   *41*

    Chapter 4   Your Birth Experience   *63*

PART III   The Birthplace
              ***Hospitals, Birth Centers, and Home Birth*   83**

    Chapter 5   The Birthplace   *85*

    Chapter 6   Hospitals   *89*

Chapter 7   Birth Centers   *101*

Chapter 8   Home Birth   *115*

PART IV   Nurse-Midwife Specialties
Well-Woman Care and
Minding Your Body   127

Chapter 9   Not Just Birth: Well-Woman Care and Your
Midwife   *129*

Chapter 10   Minding Your Body   *141*

PART V   The Future of Nurse-Midwives   155

Chapter 11   The Future of Certified Nurse-Midwives   *157*

Appendix 1   Suggested Reading   *167*

Appendix 2   Organizations   *171*

Appendix 3   Educational Programs   *176*

Appendix 4   Insurance Reimbursement   *186*

Notes   *187*

Glossary   *191*

Index   *195*

❋ Introduction

T his book is a guide for women and their families who want to consider a Certified Nurse-Midwife (CNM) for their births and well-woman care. We have written it from our perspectives as a nurse-midwife, Elizabeth A. Parr, and her client, Catherine M. Poole. It touches on our relationship from the births we experienced together to counseling sessions we shared about family planning and other health issues.

As we think about changes in health care in this country, there is an increasing demand for CNMs. Nurse-midwifery care has been shown to be safe, satisfying, and cost effective. We hope our readers will have a better understanding of the nurse-midwife choice for pregnancy and well-woman care.

We start with two personal accounts of how Catherine came to choose a midwife, her birth experiences with Elizabeth, and why Elizabeth decided to become a nurse-midwife. We then proceed with detailed chapters on every aspect of nurse-midwifery care. Included here are the opinions and comments of other nurse-midwives, clients, and professionals in specialties from pediatrics to obstetrics.

This book is not a primer on gynecology and birth. If you are having a problem with your pregnancy or gynecological health, we strongly advise you to consult with your care provider.

Because some of the medical terms we use may be unfamiliar, we have provided a glossary at the end of the book. And since we don't want you to finish this book without information about where to find a midwife, birth center, and other resources, you'll find four appendixes that contain follow-up information you might need, including an appendix on insurance information. A bibliography of recommended readings and sources is also provided.

Catherine's Story

My birth experience went something like this. . . . Lounging in the birth center spa, my husband Bobby held me in his arms and we floated in the jet streams of warm gushing water. Then I felt another contraction start to rise from my abdomen. Soon it was over, and Elizabeth exclaimed, "You're doing great!" But I was so relaxed nothing seemed to matter.

Even before I became pregnant, I knew a traditional birth wasn't for me. I had always been dismayed by my mother's experience in the 1950s of never seeing even one of her five newborns arrive because she was knocked out with ether. I also wanted to avoid the modern experience of my older sisters: being attached to monitors and IVs and given enemas, epidurals, and episiotomies in a hospital.

Hospitals make me tense up from the atmosphere of sick people and the smell of antiseptics. I started to question why a normal, healthy event such as having a baby needed to happen in a hospital, especially since so many generations before us were born at home.

Then I heard about a birth center from friends at work. I decided to visit it. It was staffed by CNMs, and it sounded as if it was the alternative I was looking for, although I really wasn't sure what a midwife was and worried about whether midwifery care was safe. I decided to schedule my next annual gynecological exam there, which I had heard the midwives provided in addition to prenatal care.

During my time at the birth center, the midwife and I talked about everything from family history to each of my health concerns. She was bright and caring. When she took my blood pressure it was lower than ever before. I'm convinced this was a result of the relaxing atmosphere, since my pressure was always low (100/60 or less) on subsequent visits, whereas at my doctor's it was 120/70 or higher. Although my obstetrician/gynecologist was a warm and gentle man, I was always rushed in and out to see him after waiting an hour or more in a crowded waiting room. It always seemed his time was valued and mine wasn't.

When it was time for my internal exam and Pap smear, the midwife warmed the speculum in tepid water and apologized because her hands were cold. During the exam she explained to me exactly what she was doing. She asked if I felt any discomfort and warned me if she thought she might create some. I'd never been so relaxed during this dreaded exam. Yes, this was where I wanted to have my baby and all my reproductive health care.

A year later I was pregnant. I actually enjoyed going for my prenatal visits. The midwives were like best friends and therapists rolled into one. We were on a first-name basis from day one. The nurse-midwives seemed personally involved with me, my husband, and my baby-to-be. Yet they still maintained a professional attitude. I could call them anytime with the most neurotic complaint or question and they responded warmly, educating me thoroughly in their answer. Never did they imply that I was taking up their valuable time or that I was annoying (which I'm sure I was). My husband felt comfortable with them too. Although normally a quiet person, he relaxed and opened up in their presence, raising his doubts and fears about the impending birth and his role in it.

By choosing a midwife, I felt I was gaining as much control as was possible in a situation only nature really controlled. Barring complications, my birth plan was to be followed. I didn't want the use of forceps, anesthesia, or any interference that could harm my baby physically or psychologically. I also wanted the freedom to walk around or do what made me feel comfortable during labor. It was all so easy, because each of my requirements was part of the midwife philosophy too.

Of course, we were all mindful of the chance that something might go wrong. If medical interference became a necessity, I would be transferred to a hospital and the consulting physician would be called in. (This back-up is always available because all CNMs have a relationship with a consulting obstetrician and pediatrician.) But the chance of something going wrong during the birth didn't worry me, because I knew the midwife assisting me would be right by my side, even if I had to go to the hospital. I knew she'd look out for me when my husband, too emotionally caught up in the ordeal, might not be so rational or supportive. He would be free to just concentrate on us, and the midwife would deal with the hospital staff and us.

The birth center had emergency equipment on hand (although hidden away in the chest of drawers), and the building was less than a block away from a good hospital that had an intensive care unit for infants. I worried more about the baby having a problem than myself. The consulting doctor was the head of the obstetrics department at this hospital, and he told me he was very confident about working with midwifery clients. During my risk evaluation with him, which is required by most birth centers, he assured me that I was choosing a medically safe way to have a baby. He explained that only a very low percentage of women have complications at birth, and midwives provide such excellent and personalized prenatal care that their clients have exceedingly few complications.

During my prenatal visits, I was handed my chart and then would weigh myself and test my urine for sugar and mark the results. After all, it was my pregnancy, and the theory was I should get to know my body. In my hour-long appointment, my midwife asked how I felt physically and mentally, and she provided solutions to any problems I was experiencing. She educated me about the baby's development and what he or she looked like at each stage. I met each midwife on staff and got to know them all personally. Any of them would be great to have at the birth. But there was one I felt especially comfortable with: Elizabeth. I asked if she could be there for the birth, and she said she would try. I could have my baby how and where I wanted, and with whom I wanted. I felt increasingly empowered rather than frightened of this venture.

I had a say in everything. I was even given the option of keeping the placenta and taking it home to bury in the garden— but decided against the idea since my dog would probably dig it up. Anyone within reason could come to the birth. If I had other children, they were welcome as long as each one had an individual support person. Jesse was my first child, and since I feel birth is a private thing, I just wanted to be alone with my husband and midwife.

Everything went smoothly during my pregnancy until the latter part when I was sure the baby was no longer moving. I called the midwifery center on a Saturday and they said to come right in and a midwife would meet me to do a nonstress test. Using a fetal monitor, they watched the heartbeat pattern for a while to make sure everything was normal. (A stress test, on the other hand, is when pitocin, the synthetic hormone that stimulates contractions, is administered and then the baby's heartbeat is monitored to see how it handles the stress of minor contractions.) It turned out that the baby was fine—I probably just had first-time-mother's jitters. But instead of patronizing me, the midwives took my concerns seriously. They often indicated that I knew what was going on with my body and that they trusted my intuition.

When my due date came and went the midwives were not concerned. They said the baby decides when to come and just wasn't ready yet. I had no genetic prenatal testing or ultrasound, but Elizabeth estimated that the baby weighed about 8 pounds. (She was off by just 1 ounce—Jesse weighed 7 pounds, 15 ounces!)

As it always does, the day of birth came. I was exactly a week late. When I started bleeding a little and had mild cramps, I called the birth center and the midwife told me to relax and call if the contractions changed in intensity. "Eat heartily, go for a walk, stay busy" was their advice. So I planted a peach tree for my baby and worked around my garden the rest of the day. I was too excited to rest. At about seven that evening the labor pains became much worse and I started feeling anxious. The midwife's advice was to drink a glass of wine and go sit in the bathtub. So I did and immediately felt better—until I got out of the tub.

Around midnight the contractions were getting pretty close, and Bobby was becoming exceedingly nervous. We called to say we'd be at the birth center in an hour, and to please ask Elizabeth to be there.

The labor pains became much worse in the car, and there was no room in our subcompact for getting comfortable or finding distraction. I thought the situation could be likened to being required to stay in a hospital bed strapped to a fetal monitor and IV. I was really starting to lose my cool, urging Bobby to run traffic lights. His nervousness turned to panic: He was sure I was going to have the baby in the car. Needless to say, we arrived at the birth center feeling stressed but with plenty of time before our baby arrived.

Elizabeth was there to greet us. As I walked into the birth center door I had a powerful contraction and started crying. Elizabeth rubbed my back until the contraction subsided, and her presence soothed both of us immediately. We settled into our room while she filled the spa for us. She checked me internally to see how I was doing. My cervix was dilated only 4 centimeters. I was discouraged; I had endured all that pain for so long and wasn't even halfway dilated. As soon as the water was ready we eased into the spa and we both relaxed. After about 40 minutes in the tub I felt like pushing and believed I was definitely in transition (the period of labor usually prior to pushing). Elizabeth seemed skeptical that I could be that far along already.

We moved to the bedroom from the tub and she checked me again. I was 8 centimeters or more dilated. In just 40 minutes at the birth center I had made more progress than I had all day and night at home. I was only 2 centimeters away from the magic number of 10, when I would be ready to push. Elizabeth decided to help the last bit along, since I was becoming exhausted. She gently nudged my cervix and all of a sudden Jesse was on her way down. Elizabeth ran to put on her green scrubclothes and told me not to push yet.

Normally a registered nurse (R.N.) assists with the birth, but this time it was quicker to get one of the other midwives who was there and on call. I felt totally spoiled by the attention of two midwives. I lay on my side on the double bed with Bobby up by my head. Shelly Grubb, the other midwife (who later attended Elizabeth's birth!) was on the other side of Bobby. Elizabeth was between my legs. Shelly gave me sips of Gatorade® to keep my strength up as well as lots of encouraging words. I gave a big push and accidentally kicked Elizabeth right off the bed. With another push I pulled Bobby's sweat pants down to his knees.

The midwives positioned a mirror for me to see the baby coming. Elizabeth said there was a lot of dark hair on my baby, but I thought she was just trying to make me feel better about the baby being so close. But in a flash our daughter was lying on my stomach. Bobby helped cut the cord after it stopped pulsing. We named our new little girl Jesse, for her great grandmother, Jesse Virginia.

They wiped Jesse with towels and wrapped her to keep her warm, and she started nursing right away. Then the midwives quietly disappeared into the family room, close by, yet unobtrusive. We called our mothers and a few other people and then stared some more at Jesse. The three of us dozed a little and then ate some snacks. In a few hours it was time for Jesse's physical exam and weighing in. I was tired, but felt wonderful otherwise. Four hours after Jesse was born we were ready to go home. Birth centers all differ in their discharge policies, but normally they'll send you home 4 to 12 hours after the birth if everything is stable with you and the baby.

Then Elizabeth gave us instructions for the next few days. We would be taking Jesse's temperature and pulse as well as my own every 4 hours. I was not to emerge from my bed for two days. Bobby was to feed me well. The birth center's nurse, an R.N., would come to our house in a few days to see how we were doing and to perform the PKU test on Jesse (a routine blood test for a metabolic disorder).

As we walked out to the car I held Jesse in my arms while Bobby helped hoist the flag over the midwifery center, proclaiming "It's a Girl!" Driving home was strange, because there in the back seat was a tiny baby in the huge car seat that rode empty just a few hours before. At home we all fell exhausted into bed. I was too excited to sleep and just wanted to stare some more at Jesse. She was sleeping with her hand under her chin, exactly like her dad. I wondered if sleeping positions were genetic.

At two weeks, Jesse had her first glimpse of a doctor, her

pediatrician. He commented that the babies he sees delivered by CNMs rarely lose weight in the first few weeks whereas hospital-born babies lose a pound or so. Jesse had gained 8 ounces since birth. He was also impressed with the thorough physical exam given Jesse by the midwives. And Jesse was, to quote the pediatrician, "in perfect shape."

My second baby, Carey, a 10 pound boy, was quite a different story. He was born on Jesse's birthday, for which I will always blame Elizabeth. Elizabeth worried that he was getting too big and that I would have a tough delivery if he kept gaining weight each week. So the day before he was due she did something called "stripping the membranes," which she explained is done by stretching the cervix during a pelvic exam. That night my water broke, although labor didn't begin until morning. We left home with a few easy contractions, and in the 45 minutes it took us to get to the birth center I had skipped through transition to full dilation. Although the labor was short, it was more intense, and I was thankful for Elizabeth's gentle guidance and reassurance through each contraction. I had a lot of plans to do what I hadn't done the first time, but I barely got to stick a toe in the spa before pushing my son Carey out in record time.

Three year-old Jesse wasn't there for the birth. But Laura, a special friend, brought her to the birth center an hour later. Jesse waded through the crowd of visiting midwives. She hopped up on the bed and proudly held her brother, giving him lots of kisses. We left the birth center only a few hours after the birth since we were in excellent shape and anxious to get home to be a family alone together. We drove home this time with Jesse and Carey sitting peacefully together in the back seat.

Each time I couldn't have asked for a better family birth. The midwives allowed me to have two birth experiences that I will always look back on, smiling. I believe our family's bond is stronger, and I'm thankful for the midwives' guidance in teaching us to take responsibility for maintaining our health. I will always thank my lucky stars (my mother's expression) that I chose a nurse-midwife.

Elizabeth's Story

Catherine and I met when she came to the birth center for a well-woman exam, long before we decided to write this book. Like many of our clients, she was seeking an alternative to conventional women's health care. She wanted a more personal relationship with her caregiver and more involvement in the care she received. And these were the same compelling reasons I became a midwife—to provide this kind of satisfying health care to women.

I first heard about midwifery when I was a senior in college, finishing a degree in French. One of my housemates came home one day and announced she was going to become a midwife. To me, the word conjured up images of medieval childbirth or old southern "grannies." So I was intrigued by the chance to go with my friend to visit a nurse-midwife who practiced in a low-income clinic several miles away.

I had no idea what to expect. We were greeted by a warm and friendly woman in her forties, dressed conservatively, who turned out to be a nun. During our visit she explained that she was a CNM. As we talked, I was impressed by her professional manner and the extent of her knowledge of the field. She was clearly an important part of the medical system, and yet I sensed something different.

We gained a lot of information that day, but what I remember most vividly was the interaction I observed between her and one of her patients, a young woman whose baby she had recently delivered. I sensed she had made a big difference in the experience of this apparently underprivileged young mother. They chatted intimately, and I could see the midwife really cared as she cooed and gurgled at the new baby. I'd never experienced that kind of feeling with any health-care professional, and it struck me that this was the way it should be, especially for such a personal experience as giving birth.

Driving back to our college town, I felt a growing sense of exhilaration. I'd just been exposed to what might be a meaningful and fulfilling career for me.

That was in 1976. Although my friend never did become a midwife, I spent the next several years pursuing that goal. This meant obtaining a nursing degree and several years' experience in maternity nursing and meeting as many midwives as I could along the way. For example, during nursing school I found a job at a birth center staffed by nurse-midwives. I feel lucky that the first birth I ever saw was in such a wonderful setting. It was very different from the tense medical dramas I'd seen on television or even from what I'd been taught in my obstetrics course in school. I was awed by the nurse-midwife's ability to gently guide the couple through the birth while respecting that the experience belonged to the family, not her. Afterward someone asked me if I were the woman's sister, probably because tears were streaming down my face. I've been in love with birth ever since.

In 1984, I graduated from the University of Pennsylvania's graduate program in nurse-midwifery. Since then I have practiced primarily in a freestanding birth center, but I have also worked in hospitals and family planning clinics and have attended a few home births. During these years I have repeatedly found myself explaining my profession to people who have never heard of a "modern" midwife. The same questions have popped up time after time, and many women have expressed their dismay that they missed out on midwifery care—sometimes because they weren't aware it was available and sometimes because they had misconceptions about the safety and benefits of such care. It is for women and families like these that we decided to write this book.

Since we started this project I have given birth to my son
Sam, with the support of my husband Ed and my good friend
Shelley Grubb, CNM. This experience only strengthened my interest in spreading the word about midwifery care. All women
deserve to have as positive a birth experience as I had, thanks in
large part to Shelley's gentle, reassuring guidance and skill. It is
our hope that all women will become educated about nurse-midwifery and that this option will be available for all who choose it.

PART I

Nurse-Midwives and Clients

1

Choosing a Nurse-Midwife

As a nurse-midwife and midwife client we want you to know everything there is to know about the family-centered health care midwives offer women. In this chapter we explain how midwifery has evolved over the years to what it is today. We discuss the educational background of midwives, the scope of their practice, their philosophy of care, and the relationship between nurse-midwives and physicians.

Nurse-midwives and physicians

At first glance you'll see a lot of similarities between the care administered by an obstetrician/gynecologist and that by a CNM. Both practitioners evaluate you for the same physical problems that occur either in the gynecological aspects of your health or in your pregnancy, and both have access to much of the same medical technology. When you take a closer look, however, there are significant differences between the two types of caregivers.

Physicians are specialists in medical complications that are likely to require technologic intervention, whereas midwives are experts in normal maternity and well-woman care, seeking to remedy problems through a natural approach. By working together as a team, physicians and midwives offer women and their families the best of both worlds in medical care, although at times, of course, their care overlaps.

In 1982, the American College of Nurse-Midwives (ACNM) and the American College of Obstetricians and Gynecologists issued a joint statement that supported the complementary nature of their care. Part of the statement said that "quality of care is enhanced by the interdependent practice of the obstetrician/gynecologist and Certified Nurse-Midwife working in a relationship of mutual respect, trust and professional responsibility."

As specialists in normal gynecology/obstetrics, CNMs take a holistic approach to your health care. They spend considerable time educating you about what's going on with your mind and body. By keeping you informed, your midwife enables you to take responsibility for your health, making you an informed participant rather than a passive observer. As one nurse-midwife explained, "Physicians are focused primarily on physical things. Midwives pay attention to the woman's emotional changes in pregnancy and in her general health. It's important for any woman to have these emotions dealt with by her caregivers." Your midwife gets to know what's normal for you as an individual. Best of all, a bond of trust develops between a woman and her midwife, which strengthens over time, providing the best atmosphere for good health.

What Is a CNM?

Nurse-midwives, and the safe and highly satisfying care they offer, are quickly gaining popularity in the United States. In

1990, almost 150,000 births were attended by CNMs. And women are increasingly using CNMs for their well-woman care. Despite this trend, many people are still unclear about the function of nurse-midwives.

According to the ACNM, "A CNM is an individual educated in the two disciplines of nursing and midwifery, who possesses evidence of certification according to the requirements of the ACNM."

In other words, a CNM is a health-care professional who has received advanced training to care for healthy women throughout their childbearing experiences and to provide well-woman gynecological services. A CNM provides primary care during pregnancy, labor and birth, and the postpartum period, including the immediate care of the newborn. A CNM also provides primary care to women through annual physical exams, family planning counseling, and routine gynecological care.

History of midwifery

"Midwife" means simply "with woman," and men aren't precluded from the profession. Because the majority of midwives are women (only 1 percent of CNMs are men), we refer to a CNM as "she" throughout this book.

Today's CNM is rooted in a long history of midwifery, of women helping women. For centuries women have been attended by other women during childbirth. These traditional midwives supported and nurtured women through birth, viewing the birth of a child as a healthy event of life. They had a relatively good safety record in the years when little was known about obstetrics. The *American Journal of Public Health* reported in February 1913 that midwives, in fact, often had better outcomes than the physicians of their day. This record was probably due in large part to their philosophy of letting nature take its course, as opposed to the approach of physicians, who with little formal training attempted to control birth by such interventions of their time as bloodletting, forceps delivery, and use of chloroform.

Midwives were largely replaced by physicians in the United States by the beginning of the twentieth century. In 1900, half of the births in this country were attended by midwives; by 1930, the number had dropped to 15 percent. There were a number of reasons for this gradual demise of traditional midwifery, including the lack of access to training for midwives, the development of hospitals as the birthplace, and an antimidwife campaign by physicians.

Most early midwives were immigrant women or southern "grannies" who had little or no formal training. Although a few efforts were made to organize and educate midwives, these were considered temporary measures until physicians could take over. However, the physicians generally weren't much better off: A 1911 study by J. Whitridge Williams of the Johns Hopkins University School of Medicine revealed that most medical students had never delivered a baby by the time they graduated and that one quarter of the medical schools admitted their graduates were not competent to practice obstetrics. In fact, midwives continued to lose fewer mothers than did physicians. A study done by the New York Academy of Medicine and published by the Commonwealth Fund showed that from 1930 to 1932 the death rate for patients of midwives in New York City was much lower than that for women under the care of physicians. The White House Conference on Child Health and Protection of Fetal Newborn and Maternal Morbidity and Mortality supported this finding in a 1933 release (published by The Century Company).

The next factor affecting the practice of midwifery was the moving of the birth site from women's homes to the hospital, starting at about the turn of the century. Midwives, who had always delivered babies at home, didn't have access to hospitals. Now, more and more women sought hospital births as physicians convinced them a hospital was the only "safe" place to be. However, contrary to popular belief, mortality rates did not improve as a result of this move. In fact, a 1918 study by the federal Children's Bureau revealed that the United States had among the highest rates of infant and maternal mortality in the industrialized world.

In response to these bleak findings, major efforts were made to improve the quality of medical education and hospital care. Unfortunately, many physicians reacted by blaming midwives for the high maternal and infant mortality rates, despite ample evidence to the contrary. Much was written about the "midwife problem" and the need to view childbirth as a dangerous and complicated medical procedure best handled by physicians.

As a general rule, midwives of this era were not sophisticated. Many were uneducated, poor, and isolated from one another. As a result, they were unable to defend themselves against these accusations, and their numbers continued to decline.

Then, in 1925, the first nurse-midwives were introduced to the United States from Great Britain. They were recruited by Mary Breckenridge of the Frontier Nursing Service, who sought to improve the care of poor Appalachian women and families in her native Kentucky. These midwives have gone down in history for their dedication and bravery, traveling on horseback throughout this inaccessible mountain region with their supplies stuffed in their saddlebags. They retained the noninterventionist philosophy of the traditional midwives but had the added benefit of education and training, which allowed them to recognize complications when they occurred and to intervene when necessary. As a result, the maternal and newborn death rates in this region dropped lower than the rate for the state of Kentucky as a whole and lower than that for the entire United States.

The Frontier Nursing Service sent U.S. nurses to Great Britain to train as midwives until the outbreak of World War II. In 1939, it started its own educational program, which continues to educate CNMs today. Earlier, in 1931, the first U.S. nurse-midwifery education program was founded at the Lobenstine Midwifery School in New York City. This and several other programs were developed to meet the needs of poor women in areas around the country with limited access to care, but the number of nurse-midwives was still very small.

In 1955, the American College of Nurse-Midwifery (now the ACNM) was incorporated as the professional organization for CNMs. Since then the number of nurse-midwives has increased dramatically. There was a 500 percent rise in the number of hospital births attended by CNMs from 1975 to 1987. While over the years CNMs have continued to work extensively with poor women, during the 1970s a new group of women discovered the benefits of midwifery. Many educated middle- and upper-class women, disgruntled with the traditional medical system that viewed birth as an illness, sought a more personalized birth experience through midwifery. In response, CNMs started to open private practices and freestanding birth centers, where these new clients were able to participate more actively in their health care.

Today's CNM

Today over 4,500 CNMs practice in all 50 states, attending women from all walks of life. Nurse-midwifery practice settings range from high tech urban hospitals to health maintenance organizations (HMOs) to birth centers to women's homes. The clientele ranges from highly educated professional women to young teenagers and from very poor women to very affluent ones. Such celebrities as Susan St. James and Cybil Shephard have used CNMs, as have immigrants from Third World countries. Some CNMs maintain their own practices; others are employed by hospitals, clinics, physicians, HMOs, or other CNMs. However, all CNMs share certain characteristics.

Education

To become a CNM, one must attend an ACNM-accredited educational program. Currently there are 36 such programs for nurse-midwives in the United States (see Appendix 3 for list). To be eligible, a student must first be a registered nurse, usually with experience in obstetric, gynecologic, and/or public health nursing. Programs range from nine months to two years in length, depending on the type: Some award master's degrees while others just grant certification. There are also a few "precertification" programs designed for foreign-trained midwives seeking U.S. credentials.

A student nurse-midwife receives advanced education in all aspects of health care to women and newborns, including the handling of medical complications and high-risk situations. Nurse-midwifery programs also offer a variety of other courses in such areas as ethics, health and wellness, family theory, professional issues, research methods, communication, and pharmacology.

In addition to this theoretical course work, a student nurse-midwife spends extensive clinical hours attending women under the supervision of faculty members. Upon completion of the program, a student is eligible to take the national certification exam administered by the ACNM. After successfully passing the exam, she becomes a CNM.

Each CNM must meet her state's licensing requirements. In addition, the ACNM requires that a CNM maintain competency by participating in continuing education. The ACNM also mandates peer review, whereby all CNMs are evaluated by their peers every few years to ensure the quality of their care.

Midwifery in Canada

The practice of midwifery in Canada has not been regulated until now, but many of the provinces are actively working toward or have already developed legislation governing midwives. Although the specifics vary from province to province, it appears that midwifery in Canada will be an autonomous, primary-care specialty, separate from either nursing or medicine.

The first educational program for midwifery in Canada is being developed in Ontario, where midwifery was included in the Regulated Health Professions Act of 1991. Three institutions will jointly offer a "bachelor of health sciences in midwifery," with the first class having enrolled in 1993. Unlike in the United States, students are not required to be nurses. According to Karyn Kaufman, CNM, Ph.D., of McMaster University, students will undergo a three-year course, after which they will be credentialed as registered midwives by the College of Midwives.

Other provinces are watching these developments closely and are likely to move in a similar direction over the next few years. The provincial governments have recognized the contributions midwives have made in other jurisdictions and are working to include midwifery in the Canadian health-care system.

What Can a Nurse-Midwife Do?

The ACNM defines nurse-midwifery practice as "the independent management of women's health care, focusing on pregnancy, childbirth, the postpartum period, care of the newborn, and the family planning and gynecologic needs of women. The CNM practices within a health care system that provides for consultation, collaborative management or referral as indicated by the health status of the client."

In other words, a CNM manages the care of her clients independently, as long as that care remains within the scope of her practice (for more details on who is eligible for midwifery care, see Chapter 2). If a woman's course remains uncomplicated, she may never see a physician. However, all CNMs practice in some kind of relationship with one or more consulting physicians on call 24 hours a day.

A nurse-midwife is trained to perform all aspects of routine maternity and well-woman care, which include everything from administering a physical exam and Pap smear to delivering a baby. She attends preteens and postmenopausal women. She avoids medical intervention, but in cases where it becomes necessary, she is trained to administer pain medications and IV fluids, apply internal and external fetal monitors, artificially rupture the membranes, administer local and pudendal anesthesia, perform and repair episiotomies, administer medications to induce labor, and perform resuscitation. Some nurse-midwives are trained to perform more involved procedures such as colposcopy (the use of a magnifying instrument to examine the vagina and cervix for abnormalities) or using a vacuum extractor to deliver a baby.

Along with these technical skills, nurse-midwives are particularly skilled at counseling and educating their clients. They are well informed about nutrition, childbirth preparation, breastfeeding, sexuality, and alternative therapies. They are experts in supporting women through labor and in using nonmedical techniques to hasten and ease the birth process. Their care emphasizes prevention of complications through careful screening and patient teaching.

One new mother who was attended by nurse-midwives said,

> Although my labor and birth were relatively easy, I couldn't get my baby to nurse after I got home. I was at my wit's end, feeling like a complete failure as a mother, when my husband called the midwives. One of them actually came out to my house and helped me to get the baby to latch on correctly—and that was all it took. I guess I just needed a little extra support, because from then on we did fine.

The Midwife Philosophy

Midwives retain the with-woman philosophy of care today: They are "with" women as they listen to their questions and concerns, as they sit beside them throughout labor, and as they empower them to make informed decisions about their health.

The CNM functions within the medical system, working interdependently with other health-care professionals. At the same time, she offers an alternative to the traditional medical model, providing personalized care and addressing social, cultural, and emotional issues as well as physical concerns. She develops long-term relationships with her clients and promotes the involvement of family members.

The midwife philosophy is noninterventionist. A CNM has respect for natural processes and views pregnancy as a healthy state requiring minimal intervention. She has access to the best medical technology but avoids using it unless absolutely necessary. This approach is reflected in the low rates of Cesarean births, episiotomies, and use of forceps among midwifery clientele.

The CNM believes that women are ultimately responsible for the maintenance of their own health. She encourages her clients to participate actively in their own care and involves them in decision making. She provides information, guidance, and support so they can make the choices that are best for their health care.

Catherine had just turned 36 when she was pregnant with her second baby:

> Elizabeth explained all the different types of genetic screening tests that were available, since I now had a higher chance of having a baby with a genetic problem because I was older. She also discussed what the testing would mean to us as a couple, and what we would do with the information. I felt I'd been given the information I needed in a nonjudgmental way, and Elizabeth supported our decision, for or against testing, no matter what it was.

Other Types of Midwives

In this book we discuss primarily the profession of nurse-midwifery. However, there are several other types of midwives in practice in the United States, and their status varies from state to state.

For example, some states license "professional" or "direct-entry" midwives who are not nurses but have attended a midwifery educational program recognized by the state. Other "lay" or "empirical" midwives have diverse backgrounds. They may have had formal training or completed a home study program or apprenticed with another midwife. These midwives almost exclusively attend home births. In some states they may be registered or licensed; in other states there may be no formal system of recognizing them; and in still other states they are clearly illegal.

The Midwives Alliance of North America (MANA), an organization for all types of midwives, can provide more information about non CNM midwives and their status from state to state (see Appendix 2 for how to contact MANA).

As you can see, the term "midwife" can be confusing. Many practicing midwives and nurse-midwives would like to establish one national standard for professional midwifery. Until that happens, you need to be aware of the differences between midwives so you can make an educated choice.

What to ask

As you investigate midwifery services in your area, these are some of the questions you might want to ask:

1. **What is your background as a midwife?** How long have you been in practice and in what kinds of settings? (If you are a non-CNM, What type of midwife are you? What is your training and legal status?)

2. *What is your philosophy of care?*

3. *What type of setting do you currently practice in?* If I become pregnant, what are my choices for the site of birth?

4. *Do you work with other midwives?* Will I have a chance to meet them? May I request a certain midwife, or do you share a call schedule?

5. *What is the arrangement if a complication occurs?* Who is the consulting physician? Will I have the chance to meet him or her? How does the physician's philosophy of care compare with yours? How involved will you be if I need to be referred to the physician?

6. *What requirements would I have to meet to be eligible for your practice?* What guidelines do you use to screen for risk factors?

7. *How much time can I expect to have with you at an office visit?* Will you sit with me in labor?

8. *How can I reach you in an emergency?* What if I just have a question?

9. *What are your fees, and are they covered by most insurance plans?*

10. *What are your expectations of me?*

Why Choose a Midwife?

Nurse-midwifery care is an option that may not be right for every woman. However, more and more women are choosing CNMs as their health-care providers for many reasons.

Jane Brody, personal health columnist for the *New York Times,* told us,

> As far as patient care is concerned, it's been my observation that the vast majority of women having babies would be hard put to do better than to have a nurse-midwife taking care of their maternity care and birth. I know couples who could afford, or whose insurance would cover, the cost of an expensive obstetrician. But they weren't concerned about money. They were concerned about having as comfortable and natural a birth experience as possible, and that's what they achieved with a CNM.

Nurse-midwives are highly trained professionals, and, as we discuss in Chapter 2, they provide very safe care. Their services also cost less than traditional medical care. They are particularly knowledgeable about health-care alternatives and are skilled in the art of listening. However, most consumers who choose this option do so because they are looking for a more personalized experience in which they are treated as individuals and are encouraged to participate actively in all decisions.

As Catherine explained, "I chose a midwife because I wanted someone who would be willing to spend the time to explain things to me in language I could understand, and who wouldn't take offense if I had my own opinions about things."

Women who have used nurse-midwives indicate that they are highly satisfied with the care they received. In 1985, the Institute of Medicine reported that women who use midwives are more likely to keep appointments for prenatal care and to follow treatment regimens than women who are not attended by midwives. In a 1986 evaluation of CNMs and other nonphysician providers, the Office of Technology Assessment found that women are particularly pleased with the interpersonal aspects of the care they receive from CNMs.

Don Creevy, a practicing obstetrician/gynecologist in Portola Valley, California, and Clinical Assistant Professor of

Obstetrics/Gynecology at Stanford University School of Medicine, said:

> I have supported, worked with, and provided back-up for nurse-midwives since 1968. I have done this because I firmly believe that low-risk pregnancies and births are best handled by midwives who are backed by obstetricians and hospitals, and because I think women giving birth should have a free choice for the place of birth and attendant. CNMs provide more humane care than most physicians, with a stronger emphasis on nutrition and the psychological aspects of health.

In the following chapters we discuss more about the care provided by a nurse-midwife and its advantages. For now, midwifery is perhaps best described by the words of a woman who gave birth with a CNM: "Most obstetricians say they 'deliver' babies. Midwives say they 'attend' births; it is mothers who deliver babies."

2

Can I Go to a Midwife?

Chances are, you will have no problem qualifying to have your baby or receiving well-woman care from a midwife. In this chapter we explore who can be a midwife client and what happens if her health or pregnancy becomes at risk.

The Midwife Client

Generally speaking, most women of childbearing age are healthy and are unlikely to experience serious problems with pregnancy, labor, and birth. Unfortunately, many consumers don't realize this is the case. News stories and television dramas often portray birth as a risky undertaking that requires all kinds of complicated equipment, often ending in an emergency Cesarean section to save the life of the mother and baby.

To top it off, pregnant women in the 1990s are overwhelmed

by the barrage of technology and procedures offered to them, such as genetic testing, ultrasound, fetal monitors, and epidural anesthesia. Your well-meaning friends or care providers may advise you that you are "high risk" if you are over 35 or have had a previous miscarriage or Cesarean birth. As a result, birth can become a frightening proposition. It is easy to forget that women have been giving birth for a long time and that most of them do just fine with lots of psychological support and minimal intervention.

From a medical point of view, most women are good candidates for midwifery care if that is what they choose. But even women who are at risk may do very well under the care of a nurse-midwife. History has shown that CNMs are particularly skilled in reducing deaths and illness in high-risk populations, as we saw they did in the mountains of rural Kentucky. Studies conducted in diverse areas of the country such as rural Mississippi, southern Texas, and New York City have reaffirmed that CNMs are effective caregivers for women who are at risk because of age, economic status, geographic location, and other factors.

Screening

Nurse-midwifery practices are diverse, and what is considered normal in one practice may be considered high risk in another. The screening criteria will depend upon the practice setting, the arrangements and proximity of medical consultation, local standards of care, and the skill and experience of the individual nurse-midwife.

For example, a nurse-midwife who practices in a large teaching hospital might continue to care for a woman who developed diabetes during her pregnancy, whereas a nurse-midwife attending home births in a rural area would refer such a woman to the consulting physician. On the other hand, although there are risks associated with having numerous babies, a woman expecting her tenth child in an Amish community might be considered normal, whereas her counterpart in the inner city with poor nutrition and little support would be considered at risk.

In general, nurse-midwives in independent practice and those who attend out-of-hospital births will be the strictest about whom they accept for care. Those who work next to physicians on a daily basis and in hospital settings will typically be able to care for women with more complications, since consultants are readily available. Your safety is always the first consideration.

To determine who is appropriate for care, each nurse-midwifery practice should have written policies that describe its scope. These policies should cover the criteria for acceptance into the practice and how any problems will be handled. Each potential client will be "screened" to see if she meets these guidelines. Your nurse-midwife will be happy to share these policies with you.

Elizabeth has found that sometimes women want to come to a midwife for prenatal care but are afraid that they are not eligible because of such past history as fertility problems or having had their last birth induced. She finds it nice to be able to reassure such women that these kinds of things aren't a problem and that they can get the kind of care they want.

Your screening will take place at your first visit to a nurse-midwife. She will gather information about you by taking a detailed record of your family's medical history, your occupation and family situation, your lifestyle, and your health behaviors. Along with the physical examination and testing, this information will be used to determine your eligibility and to plan your care.

After this initial screening a very small number of women will need to be referred to a physician. These are usually women with serious medical problems, such as heart or kidney disease, and in most cases they already realize they will require such care. Women with chronic medical problems like hypertension, diabetes, or drug or alcohol addiction will require a physician's involvement, but they may also receive some care from a nurse-midwife if they are in a hospital or clinic setting.

Your nurse-midwife will continue to screen you carefully at each office visit. Many nurse-midwives believe they are able to pick up problems early because they get to know their clients well and can recognize subtle changes. This ongoing evaluation of your health status will continue throughout pregnancy, labor, and postpartum and at each well-woman visit as well.

Other criteria

Along with your health status, nurse-midwives often look at other less tangible factors in determining if you qualify for their care. Your nurse-midwife may investigate such factors as your level of commitment to self-care, the extent of your support system, and your level of trust in her as a caregiver.

In accordance with the philosophy of midwifery, your CNM will expect you to demonstrate a commitment to doing what's necessary to optimize your health. Furthermore, she will expect you to participate actively in decisions concerning your care. If you are most comfortable with a pat on the head and a "don't worry, I'll take care of everything" approach, a nurse-midwife probably isn't the best caregiver for you. Your nurse-midwife considers herself to be in partnership with you to ensure a healthy outcome, and she expects you to share the responsibility.

One nurse-midwife we spoke with said:

> I attend births at home, so I need to be extra sure that my client is going to do everything she can to keep herself healthy. I want to be sure that she understands the added responsibility we each have in planning a home birth. I tell women from the start that if they can't be bothered to come to their prenatal visits or make an effort to stop smoking or improve their eating habits, then they should find another caregiver.

In other cases, you may be committed to midwifery care but lack support from your family or friends. Most nurse-midwives will encourage you to bring your doubting husband or mother-in-law to a visit, and that experience is usually enough to persuade them that your choice is a good one.

Elizabeth has been asked some very funny questions by concerned families over the years. Her favorite is, "Where's your babushka?" "I know they sometimes expect to see dirty fingernails and missing teeth, and I love to watch their looks of surprise when they meet me and realize I don't fit their image. To me, it's worth taking lots of time to reassure family members that this really is a safe choice, because I know that if family members are not comfortable, it will interfere with my client's experience."

Family support is also important to ensure adequate help at home after the birth, particularly if you opt for an out-of-hospital birth or early discharge. Your nurse-midwife will want to be sure you'll have the help you need so you can get your rest and care for the baby without other demands.

One mother of three told us, "I wanted to have my last baby in the birth center, but I knew I wouldn't have enough help if I went home the same day. The midwives attended me in the hospital, and I stayed there to rest for two days while my in-laws helped out with the other kids. I know if I'd gone home earlier, I would have been expected to do everything I normally do, and it would have been a disaster."

Finally, your nurse-midwife will want to be sure that you have trust in her as your care provider. Nurse-midwives are known for their ability to develop relationships with their clients based on mutual trust. However, some women will never feel comfortable with anyone other than a doctor. And there are a few women who want total control over decisions about their care, who don't want to share that responsibility with their midwife or anyone else. In these rare cases, a nurse-midwife will recommend care elsewhere, because the midwife doesn't want to put the woman or her baby at risk. But in the majority of cases, your trust in your midwife will continue to grow as she cares for you throughout childbearing and beyond.

What If I Have a Complication?

By careful screening and close follow-up care nurse-midwives work hard to prevent problems from occurring. In fact, nurse-midwives were praised by the U.S. Office of Technology Assessment in a 1986 report for being "more adept than physicians at providing services that depend on preventative actions."

In a small percentage of cases, however, complications do arise, sometimes unexpectedly. This is why nurse-midwifery education also includes abnormal obstetrics and gynecology, so problems are recognized quickly.

For example, a small number of healthy women develop problems in pregnancy, such as preterm labor, or perhaps discover they are carrying twins. Another small group will have uneventful pregnancies, but then experience problems in labor, such as slow progress. Others may have problems after the birth, such as heavy bleeding or a baby that doesn't breathe on its own. Many of these problems are predictable and relatively easily handled. It is rare for a low-risk nurse-midwifery client to experience a sudden life-threatening situation, but CNMs are trained to handle immediate emergencies, including resuscitation. In all cases, though, the CNM is working within a system that provides for medical consultation, so she can refer any complications beyond the scope of her practice to a physician.

Twins and breech birth

Sometimes even though you are healthy you develop a situation that requires closer watching, such as a twins pregnancy.

Although having twins is a perfectly normal event, some of your needs will be different, and you will have some additional risks. Depending on your midwife's experience and skill, and her arrangement with the physician, she may continue to care for you safely. A study of twins births conducted from 1989 to 1992 at the Medical University of South Carolina compared the outcome of the births of twins in two clinics, one headed by a physician and the other managed by a CNM. The findings revealed that the clinic run by the CNM had significantly fewer low birth weight problems and neonatal care unit admissions, as well as a lower perinatal mortality rate, than the physician-run twins clinic.

Sometimes at the end of the pregnancy a baby positions itself bottom first instead of head first. This is called the breech position. Most babies will eventually turn into the normal head down position, but if your baby is breech, your CNM may suggest that you try special exercises to encourage the baby to turn around. Or you may be referred to a practitioner skilled at "version," in which the baby is turned manually by manipulating your belly. If your baby does not turn, your CNM will advise you about what to expect at the birth. Although it is increasingly common for breech babies to be delivered by Cesarean section, some midwives and/or their consulting physicians are very skilled at vaginal breech births and may be able to offer you this option if you meet safety criteria.

The Consulting Physician

Elizabeth has found that "the nice thing about our consulting physicians is they respect our knowledge and understand we don't want to go beyond the scope of our practice. So when we refer someone, they listen carefully to what we say and discuss the plan for care. We work together very effectively."

As we discussed in Chapter One, nurse-midwives always work interdependently with a consulting physician. The nature of this relationship varies. The CNM may be the physician's employee, or she may actually employ the physician to be available as a consultant. In some cases both are employees of a larger institution, such as a hospital, a clinic, or a health maintenance organization. But in all cases the physician has agreed to be available immediately, 24 hours a day, in case a nurse-midwifery client develops a problem that requires a doctor's expertise.

This "co-management" with a physician can take several forms: consultation, collaboration, and referral. In the case of a minor problem, such as anemia (low red blood cell count) in pregnancy, the CNM may merely consult the physician, meaning she seeks the doctor's advice or opinion but maintains primary responsibility for managing her client's care. In a more complicated situation, such as a twins pregnancy, the midwife and physician may collaborate, meaning they will jointly care for the client as mutually agreed—perhaps the CNM will deliver the babies with the physician present at the birth. Finally, a client will be referred when a physician's care is required, such as a situation requiring surgery. A mother of three told us:

> I'd been going to a midwife for my annual exams for years, and I'd never needed to see the gynecologist. But last year I had an abnormal Pap smear. My midwife brought me in, explained the results to me, and told me my options. We decided that it was best for me to have further testing done by the physician she works with. Although I was scared to death, I was glad there was a physician available when I needed one. The physician was good about keeping my midwife involved as I underwent treatment, and I'm happy to say my last Pap was normal—and I'm back under the care of my midwife.

The consulting physician is someone who is qualified to practice obstetrics and gynecology. He or she may be a family practice physician, an obstetrician/gynecologist, or a perinatologist (a specialist in high-risk obstetrics). CNMs who provide care to newborns may also work closely with pediatricians and neonatologists (specialists in newborn care). In the case of a specific problem, CNMs also may consult with other specialists, from dermatologists to cardiologists. Nurse-midwives also consult with other members of the health-care team, such as nutritionists, social workers, and psychologists.

Even in the case of a complication that requires physician management of your care, your midwife may still be able to offer you support. She can help you to keep perspective on the fact that you are still a pregnant woman who will be giving birth to a baby, despite your high blood pressure or diabetes or whatever problem you have.

A 34-year-old woman who experienced infertility and two miscarriages told us:

> I knew I needed to be cared for by the infertility specialist during my first trimester because of my history. But I really didn't feel like a pregnant woman; I felt like an infertility patient. Then one of the midwives suggested I come in to see them as well as the physician. They were sympathetic to my situation (more so than the doctor, for whom my type of infertility was relatively minor), and they also gave me all the teaching and support they give everyone. It helped me to realize that even though I am an "infertility patient," I am also a pregnant woman, who is going through all the things a "normal" pregnant woman goes through.

Is it safe to go to a midwife?

Nurse-midwives have excellent safety records. Numerous studies have shown that their care can lead to a lower incidence of low birth weight, prematurity, and newborn deaths. Clients of

CNMs are also less likely to experience Cesarean sections, episiotomies, forceps deliveries, and the use of anesthesia.

As a result, several prominent organizations, including the Institute of Medicine, the Children's Defense Fund, and the General Accounting Office, have called for an increase in the use of nurse-midwives. In 1986, the Office of Technology stated that "within their area of competence . . . CNMs provide care whose quality is equivalent to that of care provided by physicians."

If you choose a nurse-midwife, you can be assured that the care you will receive is safe. A CNM is well educated, has met licensing requirements, and must keep current in order to practice. She will screen you carefully for problems and will avoid unnecessary medical intervention. She is part of the health-care team and works with other professionals to ensure your safety. But she is equally concerned that your experience be satisfying—and that is the key reason why many women seek midwifery care.

PART II

Pregnancy, Labor, and Birth

3

Prenatal Care

Pregnancy is a seemingly long journey that is best traveled with support. As you pass through each trimester new and exciting changes take place in your body. In this chapter we show you how your midwife can be a continuous source of comfort as she guides you through your pregnancy.

Preconception

If you're thinking about getting pregnant, it's not too early to visit a CNM. Midwives believe you should enter pregnancy in optimal condition, and they will provide preconception counseling to get you off on the right foot. Your CNM will advise you about what changes you should make in your current habits and lifestyle to ensure a healthy pregnancy. She will review your overall current health status and lifestyle and make recommendations accordingly.

If you're having problems getting pregnant, your nurse-midwife can provide basic fertility counseling or refer you to specialists if needed. (For more on fertility, see Chapter 9, "Not Just Birth.")

Some midwifery practices offer complimentary group or individual sessions in which they provide information about their services. This way, you can determine whether their practice and facilities meet your needs even before you become pregnant. Women are often pleasantly surprised to find a midwife will spend so much time with them even before they have conceived.

The First Trimester

The first trimester consists of the first 13 weeks of pregnancy, and ideally your first visit should take place during this time. This first prenatal visit is lengthy, sometimes lasting up to two hours. If you're not familiar with CNM care, the midwife will explain her credentials and the nature of her practice. She'll answer thoroughly any questions you have and will make sure you understand the answers. In this and subsequent visits she'll encourage you to ask questions, no matter how trivial you might think they are. One nurse-midwife client told us, "I was always too intimidated to ask my doctor a question. I was amazed when my nurse-midwife listened to my concerns. I never hesitated to ask her a question after she said to me, 'The only stupid question is the one you don't ask!'"

Your history

As we discussed in Chapter 2, your nurse-midwife will screen you to be sure you're a good candidate for her practice. She will take a detailed medical history, family history, and history of previous births. She will ask many questions that will help her to determine how far along you are, such as when your last menstrual period was, whether it was normal, what symptoms of pregnancy you're experiencing and when they started, and whether you know when you conceived.

One midwife client explained:

> I went to a midwife for the first time with my third pregnancy. Although I'd had wonderful birth experiences before, I noticed a difference at the very first visit. With my first two babies I told my physician I was due 10 days later than the date he gave me, because I always know exactly when I ovulate, and my cycles are long. But he went by the book, and, of course, both babies were called "overdue." But during this pregnancy the midwife listened to what I had to say, and even wrote the date I told her we'd conceived on the chart. My baby came just when we expected it, and it was nice that my midwife respected that I knew my own body.

After taking your medical history, your nurse-midwife will dig deeper into your background. She'll question you about your use of medications, recreational drugs, alcohol, and cigarettes and whether you have had any exposure to other potentially harmful agents such as chemicals and radiation. She'll ask about your work life, dietary habits, and exercise routines. She'll explore your social background and family life. She may ask whether the pregnancy was planned and how you feel about it. She will ask about your relationship with the baby's father and who will be helping you to raise this baby. She may ask about siblings and other family members and how they feel about the pregnancy.

In asking these questions, your CNM is not trying to pry into your personal life, but instead is continuing to screen you for potential problems in your pregnancy. She knows that your level of commitment to having a healthy pregnancy and your social support system play major roles in how your pregnancy proceeds. She also understands that pregnancy and birth are significant events in your life, and she cares about how you are handling these changes.

The examination

After you finish discussing your personal and medical history, you'll undergo a thorough physical exam, from head to toe, including a Pap smear. One of the important things your midwife will check is the size of your uterus, which helps her to confirm how far along your pregnancy is. She doesn't rush through the exam, and she explains what she's examining and why. She's gentle and treats you and your body with dignity. She reassures you and warns you if what she does might cause some discomfort.

Testing

Along with the history and exam, your CNM will request some lab work, including a urinalysis, tests for blood type, Rh factor, antibodies, and syphilis, and a complete blood count. These standard tests in pregnancy are done to rule out possible problems such as infections, blood incompatibility, and anemia. Additional tests for exposure to sexually transmitted diseases, German measles, tuberculosis, toxoplasmosis, and the AIDS (HIV) virus may be recommended, depending on your history. The midwife will thoroughly explain every test and then interpret the results for you. A nurse-midwife client said, "My midwife took blood from me in her office. During the procedure she said, 'I don't like drawing blood from you, but today we have to do this to find out—and then she explained the exact nature of the test and how the results were important for me and my baby's well-being."

During your first trimester, your CNM will discuss with you other tests and procedures that may be offered during your pregnancy. You should have access to any of these that are commonly available, but your nurse-midwife will help you to understand and/or decide which ones are right or necessary for you. In general, nurse-midwives do not routinely recommend prenatal tests but will not hesitate to order them if there is a medical indication.

For example, women who are at risk for genetic abnormalities because of age or family history are offered genetic testing. Your CNM will tell you what testing procedures are available to you (usually amniocentesis or CVS—chorionic villus sampling; see Glossary), the risks involved, and what information you can and cannot gain from such testing. Her role is to provide basic information and to help you explore your feelings so you can make the decisions that are right for you. If you are interested, your midwife will refer you to a genetic counselor for further information. If you choose to undergo any of these procedures, you will be referred to an experienced physician.

Sometimes an ultrasound (also called a sonogram or scan) is recommended in pregnancy. This test can provide useful information, particularly if there is any confusion about how far along you are or if you experience certain problems such as bleeding or abnormal growth of the baby. Although ultrasound is generally believed to be safe and is frequently routine in traditional medical settings, your CNM may or may not feel that there is a medical indication for you to have one.

A recent study has found that giving routine prenatal ultrasound wastes more than $1 billion a year and that 80 percent of all mothers-to-be are at such low risk that they don't need ultrasound unless problems arise. The six-year, $7 million study, completed in August 1993, is the largest to examine ultrasound benefits in pregnancy and was financed by the National Institute of Child Health and Human Development. If an ultrasound is recommended, your midwife will explain to you exactly what information she hopes to receive and why it is important. Some nurse-midwives are trained to perform the ultrasound themselves, but in many cases you will be referred to a physician or diagnostic center for this procedure. You should feel free to discuss this and any other procedure with your midwife so you are comfortable with it before it is performed.

Diet, exercise, and employment

The rest of the visit is spent sitting and talking some more. During this and future visits, your CNM will provide information about what to expect physically and emotionally during your pregnancy and will advise you on how to ensure the healthiest pregnancy possible.

Since good nutrition is vital for a healthy pregnancy, your midwife will ask for a complete rundown of what you eat daily. She will talk to you about normal pregnancy weight gain and if needed will suggest ways to improve your diet. She knows that every woman's body is different, and she is more concerned about the quality of the food you eat during pregnancy than simply the number of pounds you gain. She is also sensitive to body-image issues, which many women face. A nurse-midwife client told us, "I was overweight going into my pregnancy. The midwife took a lot of time to discuss this problem with me. She asked me to detail everything I ate in a given day. When I told her I liked to binge on junk food, she said OK, eat sensibly six days, and then on Sunday you can have a pig-out day. But I'll bet you won't miss the junk food after a while."

CNMs know that moderate exercise is important to a healthy pregnancy. Your midwife will discuss with you your current level of exercise and how to modify it for the pregnancy if necessary. If you're not very active, she'll advise you about what kind of exercise is safe to start during your pregnancy—usually low-impact activities such as swimming or walking.

If you are employed, your CNM will also discuss your work plans for the pregnancy and afterward. She'll give you practical advice about how to balance your job with leisure activities and how to get enough rest to keep yourself in good condition during the pregnancy.

In case of a problem

Your nurse-midwife will make sure you know how to reach her, day or night, and will urge you to call anytime you have a question or concern. She will inform you of the type of arrangement she has with her consulting physician or physicians, who are available 24 hours a day, 7 days a week, for any questions or complications that arise during your pregnancy. In some cases, nurse-midwives work with more than one group of physicians, and you are given a choice of which group you prefer.

In most midwifery practices you will meet with the consulting or staff physician at one of your visits. This gives you the chance to ask questions about how they will be involved in your care and to get some sense of their approach. In many cases you will never see the physician again, but you are reassured to know that he or she is there if needed.

Along with the normal symptoms of pregnancy, your CNM will educate you about the warning signs of serious problems that can occur. Probably the most common problem in the first trimester is vaginal bleeding, which may or may not be serious. Your CNM will want to hear from you immediately if you experience any bleeding so she can determine whether there is a problem. She understands how frightening bleeding can be, and she will take as much time as she needs to get a clear picture of what is happening and to make sure you have the support you need. One client who experienced this problem told us:

> I had some spotting of blood when I was six weeks pregnant. I didn't want to bother my midwife, but I finally called. She explained what was going on at six weeks gestation and why spotting might be normal. She calmly gave

me plenty of information I could use to cope—because she knew what I feared. She didn't sound hurried or as though she'd said it a million times before or was doing me a favor. She gave me the gift of her time—good care is giving someone your time.

If a miscarriage does occur, your midwife will continue to play a primary role. In some cases a surgical procedure (a *dilation and evacuation,* or D & E) is necessary, and you will be referred to the consulting physician. Even so, your midwife will keep in touch with you, counseling you and your family through the grieving process. According to one client who miscarried:

> When we realized I was miscarrying, I was referred to the doctor. I felt secure and trusted this physician because she was associated with the midwives. And she turned out to be progressive and considerate of my needs. I had to have a surgical procedure, and she allowed me to have local instead of general anesthesia—something that was important to me.

The Second Trimester

During the second trimester, weeks 14 to 28, you will usually have monthly visits to the nurse-midwife. You can expect certain procedures to be followed at each visit, similar to the prenatal routines in a doctor's office. You will be asked to weigh yourself, and your urine will be tested for protein and sugar and to screen you for infections or pregnancy-related illnesses such as toxemia or diabetes. Your blood pressure will also be checked. Now your CNM will begin to measure the growth of your baby by checking the fundal height, or the distance between the pubic bone and the top of the uterus (also called the fundus). Best of all, you will hear the baby's heartbeat at every visit.

In many midwifery practices, you're encouraged to be actively involved in these procedures. Often you will be handed your chart to record your weight and with a dipstick check your urine yourself. Your partner may learn how to take your blood pressure if desired. Your midwife believes that participation in the process can help to make you feel more involved, and it reminds everyone that this is *your* pregnancy.

Nurse-midwifery practices vary widely, depending on their client load, staffing, and site of practice. But in general, you should expect a calm and relaxed atmosphere, and you shouldn't have a long wait to be seen. Because CNMs understand the importance of getting to know you and educating you, they schedule plenty of time for each visit—in some private practices, as long as an hour or more! Also, unlike physicians, midwives don't have to fit in your visit around a surgery schedule and emergencies. Of course, there is always the chance that they may be called away to a birth, but they should advise you in the beginning about how they handle such situations: Sometimes they call in another midwife or occasionally reschedule your visit.

In a large practice, the nurse-midwives usually share the responsibility of being on call for births. In these cases, you will want to get to know each midwife, so you are comfortable with whomever is on call when it's your turn. Over the course of your pregnancy, you should have the chance to develop a relationship and a rapport with each CNM. But if by the end of your pregnancy you have a strong preference for a particular midwife, it doesn't hurt to ask if she would be willing to come to your birth. If possible, your CNM practice will usually try to accommodate your wishes.

For most women, the second trimester brings more excitement and fewer physical complaints. Usually the nausea and fatigue associated with early pregnancy are resolved, and you're starting to feel really pregnant, not just "bloated." You will be

able to hear the baby's heartbeat for the first time, and will begin
to feel the first fetal movements.

Discomforts

As your pregnancy progresses, you may experience some additional discomforts. It is important to discuss any complaints with
your nurse-midwife, so you can be assured that they are normal.
Your CNM will review your symptoms with you and offer helpful
suggestions for alleviating them. She understands that although
these discomforts may be minor, relief measures that are safe
and effective will help you better enjoy the pregnancy.

Most nurse-midwives have a repertoire of nonmedical interventions to deal with such pregnancy discomforts as heartburn, varicose veins, backache, and other typical complaints of
the second trimester. Your CNM will also teach you easy and
practical ways to prevent such discomforts and to help you avoid
exposing your baby to anything that could be harmful. For example, for heartburn she will first recommend dietary changes such
as avoiding fried or spicy foods, eating small and frequent meals
rather than a few large ones, and drinking liquids between rather
than with meals. She may suggest natural remedies such as papaya enzyme or calcium carbonate and will recommend that you
avoid medications if possible. For other types of complaints your
midwife may suggest specific exercises, body positioning, and
natural remedies. Of course, at times a more traditional approach may be called for, and she is able to prescribe medications that are safe for you to take if you need them.

More testing

A few additional screening tests are offered at this stage of your
pregnancy. One is the alpha fetoprotein test (AFP) to measure
the level of AFP in the mother's blood. This test, performed be-

tween 16 and 20 weeks, determines whether your baby is at risk for certain complications, such as spina bifida (neural tube defect) or Down syndrome. Your CNM will thoroughly explain the purpose of the AFP test and the implications of its findings. For example, she will ensure you understand that if you have an abnormal result, it may be recommended that you undergo more involved testing, such as ultrasound and/or amniocentesis. She will also ensure you understand that *no* test can guarantee a "perfect" baby. She'll discuss all of these issues with you so you have the information you need to decide what's best for you in terms of testing.

Another test usually recommended during the second trimester is a blood sugar test to screen for diabetes, a condition that can sometimes occur during pregnancy. If you have an abnormal result, you will probably need to have further tests to determine if you have gestational diabetes. Mild gestational diabetes is easily managed by a nurse-midwife with careful diet and regular blood sugar checks, but at times it may become severe enough to require physician supervision. Your nurse-midwife will work with the consulting physician to manage your care in a safe manner.

Learning opportunities

Much of the time spent at your prenatal visits will be dedicated to educating you about your pregnancy and the changes you are experiencing. Your CNM will teach you and your family about the development of the fetus as you progress through pregnancy. If you have other children, they will be interested in seeing pictures of what the baby looks like at each stage. Your midwife will also teach you toning exercises, particularly the Kegel (an exercise of the muscles of the perineum, which is the area surrounding the vagina), and pelvic rocking to help prevent backache. She may recommend pregnancy exercise classes if they are available in your community. She will also start to discuss issues such as whether you plan to breast-feed or bottle feed and may refer you to breast-feeding and new parent support groups.

Your CNM will encourage you to express any fears or concerns you feel as your pregnancy progresses. She knows that pregnant women often hear "horror stories" about pregnancy and birth from others, and she wants to prevent unnecessary worries. If you are given suspicious-sounding advice about your pregnancy, be sure to check with your CNM. As one client related,

> When I was pregnant, my best friend told me I looked "awfully small," and it got me really worried that something was wrong with the baby. I told this to my midwife at my next visit, and she showed me that I measured exactly where I should. She explained that women carry differently, and you tend to "show" less with a first baby, and I was just right for my size. My midwife made me feel so much better!

Your family

CNMs regard pregnancy as a family event and welcome the participation of your loved ones. Whether your family consists of a husband and children, your mother and sister, or a close friend or lover, these persons will be encouraged to come to your visits and to get to know the midwives. They can share the excitement of listening to the heartbeat and seeing how the baby is growing.

Your midwife is tuned into how your pregnancy might affect those around you. She will be happy to answer their questions and discuss any issues of concern to them. For example, your partner may feel reassured by her discussion of the normal anxieties about parenthood experienced by many new fathers. Or she may have useful advice about coping with your older children's new feelings of insecurity or jealousy as the pregnancy progresses. She wants your family and friends to feel included and involved, because she knows that the more support you get from them, the better off you'll be.

Catherine took her two-year-old daughter to every prenatal visit for her soon-to-be born brother: "Elizabeth always made sure Jesse was involved with my exam, either helping with the blood pressure cuff or measuring my belly. She was there the first time we heard the heartbeat, and it made her feel as though she was an important part of the pregnancy. She started bonding with her brother early in the pregnancy and right after he was born, and to this day, they are very close."

Sexual concerns

Sexuality is not an easy topic for most people to discuss freely, and pregnancy brings with it new concerns. Your nurse-midwife is well informed about sexuality issues in pregnancy and will discuss these with you openly. She understands that many couples need reassurance about whether making love during pregnancy is safe, and she knows that changes in sexual interest can occur in either partner (up or down!). She can suggest alternate positions or methods of lovemaking if you are experiencing difficulties. She knows your relationship is undergoing many changes with the pregnancy and wants to help you maintain a loving relationship, which is the best foundation for healthy parenting.

One father-to-be told us:

> I didn't want to make love to my wife. We both started feeling isolated. She wanted it more than ever, while I had no sexual appetite at all. I went with her to the next prenatal visit. The midwife asked if I was afraid I might hurt the baby by entering her, which I didn't realize was exactly what I worried about. She reassured me I wouldn't hurt the baby, and soon after I felt more comfortable making love.

Complications

Although the majority of pregnancies proceed normally, your nurse-midwife will want you to be aware of possible signs of complications, and what to do if they occur. First, she will encourage you to be aware of your baby's pattern of activity (which will be different from everyone else's), since that is one of the best ways of reassuring yourself that your baby is doing well. She may teach you how to keep track of your baby's movements on a daily basis and will tell you to contact her if you notice a decrease in the baby's pattern of activity.

Your CNM will also help you to distinguish the normal aches and pains of pregnancy from more serious signs of a complication. She'll ask you to let her know immediately if you experience vaginal bleeding or leaking of fluid, or if you have cramping or abdominal pain. She will teach you about the possible problems that these symptoms may indicate, such as premature rupture of the membranes (or "breaking the water"), preterm labor, or placenta problems, including abruptio (separation of the placenta from the mother's womb) or previa (placenta implanted dangerously low in the uterus). Although she doesn't expect you to experience these complications, she knows that if you're well informed you're better able to cope in an emergency.

The Third Trimester

In the third trimester, from 28 weeks on, birth starts to become a reality. You will probably see your midwife every two weeks at this point, and in the final month you'll visit weekly. She'll continue to do the same checks of your blood pressure, weight, and baby's growth that she's done from the beginning. In addition, she will now be able to determine the baby's position by feeling your belly to locate the various parts. She'll show you where your baby's head, bottom, and arms and legs are and will teach your partner and children how to tell the baby's position, if they're interested.

A childbirth educator told us, "I can always tell which couples in my class are going to the midwives. I always ask who knows the position their baby is in, and the midwife clients are always the only ones who know!"

At the end of the pregnancy, you'll be offered a pelvic exam to look for changes that show your body is getting ready for labor. Your midwife will check your cervix to see if it is softening, beginning to open (called dilation), and/or shortening in length (called effacement). She'll also check to see if the baby is moving down further into the pelvis, which is measured by its "station," or position in relationship to the pelvic brim. She'll explain that these pieces of information do *not* tell her when your baby is coming but that they can be useful as a baseline for comparison during labor.

Elizabeth doesn't have a set routine for doing pelvic exams at the end of pregnancy: "I offer them to everyone—I find that some women, like Catherine, are eager to know if their body is undergoing changes in preparation for labor and ask to be examined every week. Other women just don't like exams and would rather put it off until necessary. I generally let the women decide, as long as there's no medical reason one way or the other."

Parent education classes

Parent education is an ongoing process during your prenatal care with a midwife. Along with the teaching she does at each visit, your CNM may also recommend that you attend parent education classes. If she does not offer her own, she will refer you to classes given in your community, usually by private childbirth education organizations, women's health agencies, or hospitals. Your CNM can advise you about which of these are best for your purposes.

At Catherine's childbirth education classes she and her husband were the only ones having a midwife attending their birth:

The teacher spent a lot of time cautioning the rest of the class about things that might happen at their births, in particular, interventions. She'd always look over at us and say, "But you are having a midwife, so you really don't have to worry about any of this happening to you." She was right. Also, I found having Elizabeth at my births, teaching me on the spot how to get through difficult contractions, was what I needed most.

For additional information, see the listing of the national childbirth education groups in Appendix 2.

Baby care

During the third trimester, you are probably starting to think of the baby as a baby. You will have a whole new set of questions for your midwife about newborn procedures and baby care. She will give you accurate medical information but will also offer good practical advice that takes into consideration your personal situation and values.

One of the first decisions you will need to make about your baby is whether you will breast-feed or bottle-feed. Your CNM will discuss with you not just the advantages of breast-feeding for you and your baby but will describe for you how breast-feeding will feel, techniques to avoid sore nipples and engorgement, and how to deal with nonsupportive friends and relatives, such as your mother and mother-in-law. She'll give advice about how to continue breast-feeding after you return to work and how to maintain your modesty if that is a concern for you. If you choose to bottle-feed, she will also offer advice and support. Although midwives are strong proponents of breast-feeding because of its myriad benefits, they are equally strong believers that each woman must make the decision that is best for her.

You may also request guidance from your midwife regarding circumcision if you have a boy. She will present the medical advantages and disadvantages of the procedure, but she understands that families don't usually make this decision based on science. She will help you and the baby's father sort through your feelings about circumcision, taking into account your cultural and religious background and personal values. If you decide you do want a circumcision done, some nurse-midwives are trained in this procedure and are able to do it for you.

In most institutions, babies routinely are given two medications shortly after the birth: vitamin K (to prevent a rare bleeding disorder) and antibiotics in the eyes (to prevent transmission of infection from the mother to the baby's eyes during birth, usually from sexually transmitted infections, which in severe cases can lead to blindness). Your CNM will review the usual procedure at your place of birth and will thoroughly explain the reasons for the medications and the side effects to the baby. If you choose to waive these medications, she'll make sure you understand the implications of doing so or if there's any particular medical concern in your case. She'll also explain the purposes of and procedure for the routine newborn screening tests (PKU for a metabolic disease called phenylketonuria, thyroid screening, and in some areas of the country, screening for additional disorders).

Choosing a pediatrician

Now is the time to look for someone to care for the baby after the birth. This may be a pediatrician, a family doctor, or a pediatric nurse-practitioner, depending on the types of caregivers available in your community and your preferences. If you aren't sure how to go about choosing a caregiver for your baby, your CNM should be able to advise you about your choices. She will encourage you to interview a variety of caregivers, because she understands the importance of finding someone you feel comfortable with to care for your baby. She may suggest topics to discuss with potential caregivers that will help you to get an idea of their level of competence and philosophy of care.

It's important to interview more than one care provider before choosing a caregiver for your baby. This is the next long-term relationship you establish with a care provider after your midwife, and it is important to find one you trust with your baby's health. Catherine found a pediatrician by asking the mid-wives at the birth center who they might recommend: "I found it was crucial to find a pediatrician who felt positively about nurse-midwives, as mine does, since he turned out to be equally sup-portive about other issues important to me such as breast-feed-ing and circumcision."

Preparing for birth

As the end of your pregnancy approaches, you will probably begin to feel your body slowing down. Your CNM will discuss with you the changes you might start to notice, such as swelling of your feet at the end of the day, increased pressure on your bladder, hip and joint aches, and a decrease in energy.

Your midwife will recommend that you balance your work with plenty of rest, since you'll have a lot of work ahead of you. She'll encourage you to spend time off your feet and on your left side, which increases the circulation to the baby and can help cut down swelling.

A CNM in a large urban practice said, "My biggest chal-lenge in the third trimester is teaching my clients to slow down and listen to their body. Career women especially seem to have a problem focusing inward instead of outward. They need to be in control. Once they can refocus their energy, relax, and let their bodies take control, they're much better prepared for labor and delivery."

During the last few months of pregnancy, you will be focus-ing more and more on the upcoming labor and birth. You may notice Braxton-Hicks contractions, which feel like a very mild tightening in your abdomen and can occur sporadically through the last few months of pregnancy. They are sometimes called practice contractions because they are not associated with labor.

Or you may even have a bout of false labor, which can feel like the real thing but doesn't go anywhere. With false labor, your cervix will not change, and the contractions usually stop when you change your level of activity.

Your CNM will explain the differences among Braxton-Hicks contractions, false labor, and true labor and how you can differentiate them. She will encourage you to call if you're not sure what you're feeling and can advise you on the best course of action. Said one midwifery client, "I came in twice with false labor before I had my baby. I just needed that extra reassurance that everything was OK, since I lived an hour away. The midwife sat with me until we were both sure it was safe for me to go home—she said she'd rather come in for a false alarm than take the chance of missing the birth!"

In preparation for birth, many nurse-midwives teach their clients "perineal massage," which is a technique that can help stretch the vaginal opening and help you avoid an episiotomy at the birth. (See more on episiotomy in Chapter 4.) Some midwives also encourage squatting exercises, which can help to expand the pelvis.

Although everyone's labor is different, your midwife will educate you about what you might expect and the signs to watch for. She will discuss ways to help yourself cope in labor and what to expect in the setting where you've chosen to give birth. Your CNM understands how excited and anxious you are about the upcoming birth and will encourage you to call as soon as you think you may be in labor.

Complications

Your nurse-midwife will continue to watch you carefully for complications. One complication that sometimes shows up in the third trimester is "pregnancy-induced hypertension," or pre-eclampsia, which is indicated by abnormal swelling, protein in your urine, and increased blood pressure. If these signs and symptoms occur, your midwife will intervene quickly to prevent the problem from worsening. Often this condition can be easily managed with bed rest and careful monitoring, but in some cases you may need to be evaluated by or even referred to the physician.

If you pass your due date, you can expect that your mid-wife will start to monitor you more closely. Whereas it is perfectly normal to give birth up to two weeks beyond your due date, there are some increased risks if you go beyond that time period. Your CNM will inform you about additional evaluations she likes to do when women become past due, which can range from simple fetal movement counts done by you each day to a thorough ultrasound examination of the baby and nonstress or stress tests (see pp. 5–6) via the external fetal monitor. She may tell you about natural techniques that can help to bring on labor if your body is otherwise ready, such as making love, nipple stimulation, and/or taking a castor oil preparation. She will advise you about when she will recommend that your labor be induced if it doesn't begin spontaneously and how and where that will be done. (See Chapter 4 for more on induction of labor.) As one midwife client explained, "My baby was two weeks late and risk entered my pregnancy for the first time. But just as in my prenatal care, there were no surprises. I was kept completely informed of what was going on with my baby and my body. My midwife also told us exactly what she planned to do if I didn't deliver soon. Luckily, the baby came before intervention became necessary." Although it is reasonable to expect that everything will go smoothly at your birth, your CNM will discuss with you now what to expect if a complication occurs in labor. She will review the role of the consulting physician and the policies and procedures that will be followed in case you need medical intervention.

Emergency childbirth

Some families travel a long distance in order to be cared for by a midwife. If distance is a concern to you or to your family, your midwife may teach you emergency childbirth procedures. Catherine's husband was concerned about this:

> I was afraid I wouldn't know what to do if Catherine delivered the baby in the car on the way to the birth center, since we lived almost an hour away. The midwife reassured me that this rarely happens—although it's publicized plenty when it does. But she took me seriously, never patronizing me. She gave us a brief course in delivery procedures. She advised bringing clean towels and a brand new pair of shoelaces to tie off the umbilical cord. She said if the baby comes in the car, "Gently help the baby out, wrap her in towels, plop her on your wife's belly, and continue on your way."

By the time you go into labor, you should be well prepared to face the challenges of giving birth and becoming a parent. Your midwife and her colleagues are there 24 hours every day to help you. You'll find it easy to call your midwife with your concerns, because by now your bond of trust has grown and is fully developed, just like the baby inside of you.

4

Your Birth Experience

For most women the birth experience is a very special life event. In this chapter we show you how your midwife is skilled to help you through labor, and birth. She will guard this experience for you, working with you to make it as comfortable and rewarding as possible.

What Will the Birth Be Like?

As your due date approaches, you will start to imagine how your birth will be. You may dream of a birth experience in which you are supported by your partner and midwife and feel strong and confident. You eagerly anticipate you and your partner holding your baby for the first time.

But at the same time it is normal and natural to feel apprehensive about labor and birth. You may be concerned about feeling pain during the birth or harbor fears that there might be something terribly wrong with your baby. You may also feel

63

trapped when you reach the end of your pregnancy because you can't turn back, as you can often do in other life situations.

You'll hear a lot of stories about what labor and birth are like. But be careful when you listen to birth stories of friends or relatives. Everyone has her own unique labor experience, and yours may be very different from someone else's. Your midwife is the best-qualified person with whom to discuss your concerns and what you can expect in labor and delivery.

No one can predict for you how your labor or birth will be. But as Elizabeth tells her clients, "If I have a sense of what you want out of this experience, either from a birth plan or conversations with you, I'm better able to individualize your care."

Your midwife will dispel many of your fears by thoroughly educating you about the process of labor and birth. Midwives know that the more they teach you about the birth process, the better prepared you'll be when the time comes to experience it. You will be educated at each of your prenatal visits. Along with the general information, your nurse-midwife will discuss the potential of having a complication and how it will be handled. She will disclose everything to you to keep you in the right frame of mind about the events that will happen rather than let you harbor fears of the unknown. Knowing the facts makes birth a much less scary venture.

You will be forming a partnership with your midwife and therefore playing an active role in your birth. This give-and-take relationship will center around your nurse-midwife giving you alternatives while you make the choices. Having input into the decision-making process empowers you, which provides an added sense of security.

One mother-to-be who switched from an obstetrician to a midwife told us:

> My first birth was with a physician in a hospital. A lot of
> things happened that I seemed to lose control over; for in-
> stance, I was given an episiotomy and Demerol. I didn't

want this to happen at my second birth, so I presented my doctor with a birth plan at my first prenatal visit. He looked at it, laughed, and said, "What you need is a midwife!" So I found a midwife, and my birth went as I hoped it would.

The Birth Plan

To help you prepare for the birth, your midwife may ask you and your partner to devise a birth plan. A birth plan puts into writing what you and your partner want or don't want to happen at the birth. Traditionally, a birth plan is a list of demands written by couples who fear loss of control over their birth experience, and is given to the doctor and hospital staff in advance so that their desires are clear to all involved. All through your pregnancy you've developed a rapport with your CNM, so she knows what you want to happen at the birth. Still, a birth plan can help surface any feelings or fears that otherwise might remain hidden. Your nurse-midwife will be happy to give you any information you need to make your own choices. You might want to consider the following questions as you plan your birth.

1. ***Who do I want with me during labor and birth?*** Will I feel comfortable with the people who plan to attend? What will their roles be? Does my partner want to cut the cord or help deliver the baby? Is that what I want?

2. ***What do I expect from my nurse-midwife during labor and birth?*** Will she be there for the entire labor? Do I want her to stay right by my side, actively involved, or do I prefer that she stay close by but in the background? Will I need the services of a doula? (See next section for information on doulas.)

3. ***How do I feel about these medical procedures: IVs,***

electronic fetal monitoring, amniotomy, pitocin, episiotomy, forceps? (See Glossary.)

4. **What positions do I prefer?** Do I want to be able to sit in water, walk around, or take a shower?

5. **What helps me best to cope with stress and pain?** Do I like to be touched? Will it help me to be able to sit in water, walk around, or take a shower? What positions do I prefer? Do I want to be distracted by conversation, or do I prefer quiet? How do I feel about pain medication or anesthesia?

6. **If I have a complication, what will my midwife's role be?** What requests do I have for the consulting physician? Who do I want with me if I need a Cesarean? What type of anesthesia do I want?

7. **Do I want to hold my baby right after the birth?** Do I want to breast-feed immediately? Do I want my baby to stay in my room or go to the nursery?

8. **How long do I want to stay in the birth center or hospital?** For home births, how long will my midwife stay with me after the baby is born? Who will help me after the baby is born?

9. **Do I want pictures or videos of labor and birth, or after the baby comes?**

10. **What other things are important to me?** What scares me?

11. **How do I picture my birth happening?**

As you think through these questions, and perhaps write down your thoughts and feelings, be sure to discuss them with your midwife and anyone else who plans to attend the birth. Your midwife will inform you about routine procedures and what your choices will be in the setting you've chosen. More important, by sharing your thoughts she will be better prepared to help you to have the birth experience you want.

Labor

Labor is just what the word implies: work. The work of labor actually starts days and weeks before the actual birth as your cervix gradually softens, thins, or effaces and in some cases starts to dilate, or open up. Labor itself is divided into three stages: In the first, as your uterus contracts, the cervix is drawn up and dilates; in the second, your body works to push the baby down through the birth canal and out into the world. The last and easiest stage of labor consists of pushing the placenta out.

Early labor

Your midwife will have taught you that labor can start in many different ways. But you will know what to watch for and when to call her if you think your labor has begun. Sometimes it's hard to tell whether what you're feeling is really labor, and if that happens, you should talk it over with your CNM. She understands the anxiety and excitement you feel and knows that reassurance at this point can go a long way toward helping you have an easier time later on.

When you call her, your nurse-midwife will spend time with you on the phone so she can get a good sense of how you're doing. She will ask you about the signs of labor you are having—

the nature of your contractions, any leaking of fluid, or "bloody show," or diarrhea or vomiting. She'll ask what you've had to eat and drink, how your energy level is, and how much sleep you've had. She'll want to be sure the baby is moving around well, too. Finally, she'll want to know how you are feeling and who is with you for support. Your midwife can tell a lot over the phone about how far along your labor is and how you are coping. She is attuned to subtle clues like your tone of voice and whether you're able to talk through contractions.

Usually your nurse-midwife doesn't feel a need to bring you in right away when labor starts. Unless she can tell from your conversation that your labor is moving quickly, you are usually better off staying at home where you'll be more comfortable. Together you will make a plan to stay in regular touch by phone until it's time for her to see you. In the meantime, she will reassure you that your body is doing all the things it is supposed to do, and she'll guide you about how to spend the next few hours until you talk again.

How you approach this early part of labor depends on your individual situation. For example, if your labor is mild and it's the middle of the night, your midwife will encourage you to go back to sleep. She may even suggest a warm bath and a glass of wine to help you unwind and to relax your uterus. If you're well rested, she may suggest that you go about your usual daily activities as long you don't do anything strenuous. If your labor isn't doing much, she may encourage you to go for a walk, which can bring on better contractions. She will also encourage you to eat lightly and drink plenty of fluids to garner as much strength as you can for more active labor.

You will want to pay attention to the pattern of your contractions so you can alert her of any changes. However, she will discourage you from counting every single contraction because it's not necessary and at this point may only increase your anxiety.

Active labor

At some point, anywhere from 1 hour to 24 hours later, you will move into active labor. In active labor, you will work harder with contractions and can no longer be easily distracted. Now your midwife may suggest you depart for your birth place. If your birth is at home, she'll join you and your family.

Your midwife will probably greet you with a smile and congratulate you for all of the work you've already done in labor. Once you've settled in, she will just sit with you for a while to assess the pattern of your labor. Then she'll listen to the baby's heartbeat, usually by fetoscope or doppler, or sometimes by the electronic fetal monitor if you are in the hospital and your midwife feels it is indicated. Although monitors are often routinely used in hospitals, a bulletin issued in September 1989 by the American College of Obstetricians and Gynecologists states that the fetoscope and doppler can be as accurate as fetal monitors in measuring fetal heart rate. Furthermore, monitors restrict your movement and can be uncomfortable. Your blood pressure, pulse, and temperature are usually checked, and your midwife will probably do a pelvic exam to see how you are progressing.

Comfort Measures. "I worked as a hospital labor nurse before I became a midwife," said a CNM who now works in a birth center. "I really believe the clients I see now in the birth centers have easier labors than the women I used to care for. It's probably a combination of more comfortable surroundings, the relationship we've developed, and the fact that I let them do what comes naturally to ease the pain of labor."

Along with this support, your midwife will show you techniques to keep you relaxed and comfortable in labor. Some women respond well to touch and are soothed by gentle stroking or by just having their hand held. Your midwife knows just the right spot to massage or apply pressure on your back and is happy to teach your partner how she does it. She may also use visualization techniques—for example, having you picture a quiet, peaceful scene you find comforting, or later on imagining your body opening like a flower so the baby can ease out.

Water can be very relaxing, and your midwife may recommend you soak in a warm tub or whirlpool or stand in the shower for a while. If you're cold, she'll bring you warm blankets and a cup of herb tea; if you're hot, she'll fan you, wipe your brow with a cool cloth, and give you sips of refreshing drinks.

Sometimes unexpected techniques to ease labor work well. One birth center keeps a game of Trivial Pursuit on hand. One nurse-midwife told us, "We've played many a game with women in active labor—I'll never forget the time a laboring mother played against three CNMs and her husband, actually won the game, and then said, 'I think I have to push.' Two minutes later, we had a baby!"

Elizabeth has found that some women are pleasantly distracted by conversation while they're in labor: "Often I've found myself asking the couple how they met, which can lead into a great conversation. It also seems to help them reflect on their relationship in a positive way as they embark on this major new adventure together. I feel honored if they share these personal stories with me."

Coping with labor is your midwife's specialty, and she'll have plenty of suggestions to help you without relying on medication. She'll maintain a positive tone while making sure you don't feel pressured to perform. CNMs know that women cope very differently in labor, and so your midwife will not treat you like every other woman. She will remind you that there are no right or wrong ways to labor. Nurse-midwives have a keen perception for matching a woman's mood and needs. This individualized approach allows your midwife to be as interactive as you need her to be with you. If being touched and massaged during contractions helps you, she'll sit right with you through each one. If you prefer to be left alone or to have your partner as your main support, she'll stay in the background, but you'll have the reassurance of knowing she's close at hand.

In most practices, your midwife will *not* leave you and your partner alone but will provide steady guidance throughout the birth process. (Unfortunately, there are exceptions—some busy midwife practices, such as in HMOs and hospital clinics, where many clients are being managed, do not allow a CNM the time to labor-sit, but instead just be there for pushing and the birth. Be sure to ask about this before choosing your midwife.) Your nurse-midwife will provide quiet reassurance that all is normal (provided it is) and will tell you you're doing a fine job. This is a team effort working toward a beautiful, relaxed, natural event rather than a tense, frantic, medical procedure.

Pain Relief. Your comfort level with where you are and who is by your side supporting you throughout labor and birth can have a profound impact on how relaxed you are. And relaxation is important in labor and birth. Medical research has shown that there is a fear-tension-pain cycle, whereby fear leads to tension, and if you are tense, you are likely to feel more pain. If you are relaxed during labor, you will tend to perceive contractions as less painful. Your midwife's presence will help allay your fears and help you achieve relaxation. Whatever her methods, your nurse-midwife is specially trained in soothing labor's difficult times.

Some women avoid using a CNM as a care provider for fear they won't be able to get pain medication if they need it. CNMs are skilled in administering pain medication and prescribe it if a situation warrants its use. Normally, pain medication is not used by CNMs as frequently as by other care providers because the extra support and comfort measures CNMs provide during labor lessens the need for pain medication.

Medication can be useful to help you relax more, to improve labor progression, or to help comfort you in a hard, prolonged labor. What your midwife offers you will depend partly on your birth site: Some midwives attending out-of-hospital births don't offer pain medication, although most have available the common mild tranquilizers and narcotics for labor. If you have opted for a hospital birth, you will have the additional option of anesthesia. The most common types of anesthesias are spinal and epidural, which numb your body from the waist down. These types of regional anesthesias are administered by an anesthesiologist or an obstetrician, but your midwife will continue to manage your labor and birth.

Epidurals are very popular but not without risk. There's no doubt they do a fine job of blocking pain while you remain awake, but they also have serious disadvantages. An epidural can lead to a longer labor because it can slow down normal labor. Because you are numb from the waist down, many times you can't push effectively, so instruments (forceps or vacuum suction) are needed to pull the baby out. A 1989 study done in Houston, Texas, on 711 first-time mothers (published in the *American Journal of Obstetrics and Gynecology*) found that Cesarean sections more likely resulted with the use of epidurals because of the slowing of labor as well as of the inability of the pelvic muscles to rotate the baby into proper position for delivery.

If you have strong feelings one way or the other about pain medication, your midwife should be aware of this beforehand. If you do request medication, she will assess whether it is a safe and advisable option for you at that point in labor. Women respond differently to medication—some get wonderful relief, whereas others just get groggy and feel a loss of control. Also, medication given at the wrong time can slow or even stop your labor.

Positions. Studies confirm that staying mobile in labor helps things to move along and to ease discomfort. Your midwife will encourage you to change your position frequently. Often you will find yourself instinctively moving into a position that feels most comfortable; at other times you may want suggestions about positions to try. Your midwife will help you find positions that are comfortable for you, such as getting on your hands and knees, lying on your side, or squatting. Some women love sitting on the toilet. Others find an idiosyncratic position that feels best.

Said one new mother, "When I was in labor I felt a lot of it in my back. Every time a contraction came, I jumped up and leaned over a dresser that was just the right height. It was the only place that was comfortable for me, so my midwife just stood behind me and rubbed my back through every contraction."

Walking continues to be an effective way to keep labor progressing. It's also helpful to give you a change of scenery, which you may need if your labor is very long. Depending on where you are, you may walk the halls of the hospital, stroll the grounds of the birth center, or even hike a nature trail. Sometimes your midwife will accompany you, and sometimes you'll take off with your partner or support person.

Elizabeth described one helpful technique that she calls the labor dance: "As the couple walks together, the woman stops for a contraction, leans on her partner, swaying her pelvis as she breathes it through."

As your labor proceeds, your midwife will remind you of other things you should be doing. She will encourage you to drink lots of fluids to prevent dehydration and may suggest you eat some light, nutritious foods to keep your strength up. She knows that this is usually preferable to having an IV in your arm, and she will order an IV only if it's really necessary. Midwives have long recognized the value of good nourishment during labor, and some have special concoctions that they recommend you drink, usually with plenty of sugar to give you extra energy.

Your CNM will also encourage you to empty your bladder frequently. In some cases, particularly in a long labor, she may even recommend that you try to rest for a while.

One mother told us:

When I was in labor with my second baby, I was overcome with exhaustion when I hit 7 centimeters and felt as though I just couldn't go on. My midwife suggested I lie down for a while. She dimmed the lights, closed the door, and sat just outside the room so she could hear me if I needed her. I woke completely refreshed an hour later and proceeded to give birth to my beautiful little girl. People don't believe me when I tell them I took a nap in active labor, but it was just what I needed.

Letting go, allowing your body to relax and do what it does naturally, is fundamental to midwife philosophy. Sometimes giving birth is compared to having sex. If you are relaxed and uninhibited, you can let go and it will be more enjoyable. Some women (who are obviously relaxed) experience sexual arousal and even orgasm during birth. Making noise, like some men and women do while making love is also a way of letting go. Many women find themselves making primal grunting or groaning noises. This groaning is very natural and can be helpful during labor, especially when you are pushing. Unfortunately, in traditional environments women may feel inhibited about making noise or having sexual feelings in labor. Most CNMs will encourage you to relax and go with the flow of your feelings.

Pushing: The second stage of labor

Many women feel a sense of relief when they are finally able to start to push (although some women don't like the feeling at all). Your midwife will encourage you to follow your instincts and push in whatever position you like, and as hard as it feels right to you. Some women need more specific guidance at this point, and your CNM can help you find an effective position. Said Elizabeth:

A client I attended was too inhibited to push effectively. I finally got her on the toilet, and like many women, she did great there. As the head started to crown, I walked her back to the bed. As soon as we got there, everything stopped again. The only way I could get her to bring it down again was by getting her back on the toilet. After a few more trips back and forth, we realized that we might as well stay put. So, with her husband supporting her, we perched her on the toilet and she pushed the baby out. I call it my "planned bathroom birth."

Pushing out a baby usually takes an hour or two, depending on whether the baby is a woman's first. Elizabeth pointed out, "You may be one of the lucky ones, like Catherine, who do it all in one or two pushes in just a short time. No matter if it's taking a long or short time, I will encourage you to do whatever works to bring the baby down." Most midwives don't demand that you bear down for a certain length of time with each contraction, which is still commonly done in traditional settings, but your CNM will give you clear guidance and instruction as you need it. Sometimes she'll bring a mirror so you can see the progress as your baby starts to crown. Or she may apply warm compresses to your perineum (the tissue that surrounds the vagina and rectum) if you find it soothing. Many midwives massage your perineum with oils to help it stretch as the baby moves down.

Friends and Family

The birth of a baby can be a wonderful family event shared by all your loved ones. You know best who you'd like to have with you, and your midwife will welcome whomever you choose. In most cases, your partner wants to be involved, but siblings, grandparents, and other close people in your life are also welcome.

Your CNM wants to meet the needs of all family members,

however you define your family. One woman shared her birth with her entire church congregation at a birth center! On the other hand, many women find birth to be a very personal and a private event, and sometimes having the wrong people there can inhibit the labor process. So it is wise *not* to invite someone who makes you the least bit uptight. One CNM said, "I've found that it's sometimes *not* a good idea to invite your mother to your birth. In many cases she is so close to you that she can't help but be anxious, and sometimes the daughter ends up comforting her mother, which doesn't help her get through labor."

If the baby's father is not involved or is uninterested in or uncomfortable with participating in the birth, your midwife will gladly accept whomever you choose to have with you, such as your sister, mother, friend, or lover of either sex.

If you don't have someone to be your support person, try asking a childbirth educator or your midwife if she knows someone who might want to help you during labor. Another great help at birth and also after birth when you're still adjusting at home can be from doulas, which is a Greek word meaning experienced women who help new mothers. For a nominal fee, these labor companions provide continuous emotional support and assistance from early labor at home through birth and the postpartum period. The service of a doula at one birth center, for example, costs $50 for the entire birth, which includes the doula doing everything from rubbing your back to walking your dog at your home. (See Appendix 2 for how to find a doula.)

The importance of having a trained labor companion can't be overstated. A study first reported in the *Journal of the American Medical Association,* and later published in the book *Mothering the Mother* by John Kennell, Marshall Klaus, and Phyliss Klaus (Addison-Wesley, 1993), studied the use of doulas in the births of over 2,000 women. The research found that a supportive labor companion shortened the duration of labor, decreased the rate of Cesarean sections by 50 percent, and reduced the need for pain medication.

Medical Technology

All nurse-midwives have access to medical technology, directly or indirectly, but generally avoid its use unless medically indicated. However, in some hospital settings midwives are more likely to use equipment like fetal monitors, IVs, and anesthesia. Some midwives work in settings in which they regularly place internal monitors, and a few are skilled in the use of the vacuum extractor.

The amount of technology you will be exposed to depends primarily on how your labor goes, but also on the policies of the institution you are in and on your individual midwife's approach. For example, some hospitals require a "baseline" fetal monitor strip, whereas fetal monitors are often not even available in a birth center. In general, the more complicated your labor and birth, the more technology you can expect to encounter. If you are not sure what to expect, you should discuss this with your midwife before your birth.

Episiotomy

Episiotomy, an incision made into the perineum, is performed when the baby is about to be born in order to enlarge the opening.

The episiotomy has been a routine procedure for many years because of the belief that it preserves the pelvic floor muscles, helps avoid tears to the perineum, and causes less pressure on the baby's head at birth.

Midwives have long disagreed with these beliefs and are expert at doing births without cutting an episiotomy. They find that even in cases where a tear occurs, it heals more quickly and there's a less painful recuperation than from an episiotomy.

A study in 1992 by the Jewish General Hospital and McGill University looked at 700 births and concurred with the midwife philosophy on episiotomy. The study concluded that episiotomies should be performed only when there is evidence of fetal distress or when instruments are needed for delivery. It also pointed out that despite the evidence against them, over 80 percent of women in U.S. hospitals still get episiotomies.

To avoid tears, your midwife will coach you to push the baby out gently as she supports your perineum. She will advise you when and how hard to push, or she may ask you to blow through a contraction so the head eases out gradually. This requires good communication skills and lots of patience, since cutting an episiotomy is quicker.

Of course, in some instances a midwife may believe an episiotomy is necessary. If she feels the baby needs to get out fast or foresees your suffering a large laceration, she is skilled at administering local anesthesia, making the incision, and stitching you up afterward.

Difficult Labors

All labors are different, and some are just plain easier than others. If you have a difficult labor, your midwife will work even more closely with you to get you through. Some labors are very long, and it is easy to become exhausted and frustrated. If you have a labor like this, your midwife will suggest ways to speed it up. Walking and alternating positions often create more efficient contractions, or she may suggest you stimulate your nipples, which releases the natural labor hormone oxytocin. If your water has broken but your labor isn't progressing, castor oil is often helpful. Castor oil stimulates the intestines, which, in turn, can irritate the uterus, starting contractions.

Your midwife will also make sure your body has enough reserves to do this work. She will urge you to keep up your intake of fluids and nourishment and will test your urine periodically to see if you're spilling ketones (which are acids that show up as you burn fat to get more energy when you are depleted of nutrients). One mother recalled her prolonged labor: "I remember them giving me spoonfuls of honey—it didn't taste so great, but it worked to give me a second wind."

Sometimes your body just needs a rest, so your midwife may suggest wine to help you snooze a little or medication to knock out the contractions long enough for you to get a break. Usually you will wake up refreshed in a good labor pattern.

And sometimes you just need to forget about labor for a while. In Elizabeth's practice, one of her best techniques to help a slow labor is sending couples out to the movies: "It helps get their minds off the labor, and usually both come back in a better frame of mind."

Most women have heard of the dreaded back labor, in which women experience most of the pain in their back because of the baby's position. Along with massage and a hot-water bottle, your midwife will recommend positions that will relieve your back pain, such as getting on all fours or switching sides or positions, and also encourage the baby to turn to another position.

Complications

Although most labors proceed normally, your midwife will be watching carefully for signs of complications. She respects the normal variations in labor and doesn't expect yours to follow any specific pattern. This flexible approach probably accounts in part for the low rates of Cesarean and forceps births in women who are cared for by CNMs. But if your midwife senses things aren't going as they should, she will act early to prevent further problems.

Sometimes a problem arises before you are in labor, and you need to have your labor induced. This may occur if you've had a complication such as pregnancy-induced hypertension or if you go too far beyond your due date. Labor may be induced by artificially breaking your water, by giving you a hormone called prostaglandin by gel or suppository in the vagina, or by administering pitocin, a synthetic form of the natural labor hormone oxytocin.

In these cases, the physician would be consulted, but your midwife may manage your labor depending on your risk status.

If your midwife recommends that your labor be induced, she will thoroughly and clearly explain why. Pitocin in particular is sometimes overused in inducing labor when there is no medical reason for doing so, but your midwife will use this intervention, like all others, only when it is justified.

Labor can proceed quickly, lasting as short as 30 minutes or lasting for days, and still be normal as long as the baby and mother are doing well. Midwives have eternal patience when it comes to long labors, but if after all of your midwife's best efforts you still are not progressing, she may suggest you boost your contractions with pitocin through an IV. Pitocin is not administered outside the hospital, so if you are not already there, you will be transferred. Your midwife will consult with the physician about starting the medication, but in most cases she will continue to care for you.

The scariest complication for women in labor is fetal distress. This occurs when the flow of oxygen to the baby is somehow compromised, which the midwife picks up from listening to the baby's heartbeat. It can occur when the umbilical cord is compressed and may quickly be remedied simply by changing the mother's position. If signs of distress aren't quickly resolved, a consulting physician will be called in, and the solution is usually to deliver the baby by the quickest means available, normally a Cesarean section. Your midwife will stay by your side during the delivery and will keep you informed of what is going on at all times.

The Birth

Finally, you reach the moment when the baby joins you and your partner. Your midwife continues to support and guide you as you ease your baby into the world. Your partner may actually assist with the birth, or you may reach down to feel your baby emerge and pull him or her up onto your body.

A midwife-assisted birth is typically quiet and peaceful. Your midwife will be carefully evaluating you and your baby right after the birth, but she does so without interfering with your first moments with your baby. There's no rush to cut the cord. After all, your baby has made a long journey out of a quiet, warm, dark place, and the outside world can be a rude awakening. You, your CNM, or your partner will cut the cord after it stops pulsing. Your baby may start nursing right away or just cuddle with you and your partner. Now your midwife will watch for signs that the placenta has separated from your uterus and will tell you to gently push it out. If you wish to examine the placenta, she'll show it to you and explain how it functioned.

Your midwife will check on you frequently to make sure you aren't bleeding excessively and that your vital signs are stable. The baby will be checked for immediate problems, and then his or her breathing, color, and heartbeat will be monitored regularly. Your midwife and her assistants will do these checks unobtrusively, so you have plenty of time for bonding. Otherwise, after you've had some time with your baby, the newborn examination is performed. Your midwife will educate you and your partner about what to look for when observing the health of your baby. She will explain what *not* to be concerned with about your baby, such as swollen nipples or hair on the back. If you gave birth in a hospital, a pediatrician or family physician typically will perform the exam. Eye drops and vitamin K may be administered to the baby with the exam.

Your midwife will stay with you for a while after the birth to make sure all is well. She will help you with breast-feeding and advise you about what to expect physically and emotionally over the next few hours and days. If you stay in the hospital, she will visit you daily. For home and birth center births, she will advise you about follow-up calls and/or visits.

Bonding with Baby

Midwives provide a very nurturing environment at birth, which enhances the bonding process. Unfortunately, some hospitals routinely separate mothers and babies. Sometimes though, even in a nurturing environment, the parents may not feel an immediate bond with their baby, and they shouldn't feel guilty, since bonding is a long-term process that strengthens over time. Pediatrician T. Berry Brazelton told us:

> The support that families need to create a nurturing environment at birth is certainly more available from nurse-midwives than from physicians. This environment is more conducive for initial bonding at birth and this bonding is important, but I don't think it is a critical aspect of nurturing later on. Bonding at birth is sometimes overemphasized, when it should be a very individualized process. There are instances where the baby has to be taken quickly to intensive care because of a problem, and the parents don't have the opportunity to bond with the baby. Or sometimes the mother needs to rest after a hard labor. Parents shouldn't feel shame because they missed immediate bonding with their baby. In these cases it has been shown that attaching to a baby takes a long time, so the magic of bonding is not just during the first moment. What is really crucial is the long-term bonding process, which takes more time and demands a greater amount of work than the first moments together. Providing support after birth is an important part of the care provided.

In this book you'll hear more than once about continuity of care. Midwives specialize in providing care from the start of your pregnancy to the finish and beyond. You can count on continued counseling and support as your CNM takes care of you and your body for many years down the road.

PART III

The Birthplace

Hospitals, Birth Centers, and Home Birth

5

The Birthplace

Many women don't give a lot of thought to where they will have their baby. They automatically assume that birth happens in hospitals with doctors because that's how they were born and how their friends had their babies. Yet, as we discussed in Chapter 1, the hospital birth performed by a doctor is a fairly recent phenomenon. In 1900, only 3 percent of births occurred in hospitals. By 1970, over 90 percent were in hospitals.

What has happened over this time period is probably best explained by anthropologist Robbie Davis-Floyd in her book *Birth as an American Rite of Passage* (University of California Press, 1992). She says, "Our birth process has been socially shaped over the years, making doctors, hospitals and medical procedures components of our birth rituals." She refers to this type of birth and the technology that goes with it as a "technocratic birth." She means that technology dictates the birth process rather than the woman and the situation at hand.

In Chapter 1 we discussed the development of the hospital as the place of birth, the reasons for this evolution, and the lack of data to demonstrate that the hospital improves outcomes for women. Although the move into the hospital initially pushed midwives out of the picture, today more than 85 percent of CNM-attended births are in hospital settings. But midwives also have been leaders in reestablishing home birth as a safe option and in developing the newest choice of birth site, the freestanding birth center.

When you choose a midwife for your birth, your choice of birthplace will depend upon where she practices. Some CNMs offer birth services in all three locations: home, hospital, and birth center. More often, CNMs offer only one or two of these options. If you're lucky enough to have several midwifery practices to choose from, you may select your midwife according to where you prefer to give birth.

According to Davis-Floyd,

> If we leave it to obstetricians to run the show, options in birth become too limited. CNMs, however, have women-centered practices, where they offer a range of options for women. And not all women want the same thing. For the woman who wants a technocratic birth, the CNM can provide that type of birth yet make the woman feel intellectually empowered. At the other end of the spectrum, the CNM offers the totally natural experience of a home birth.

Where you have your baby is important to you, your partner, and your baby. Each setting—home, hospital, and birth center—has certain advantages and disadvantages. The most critical consideration is finding the place where you and your family feel most comfortable.

Make sure you thoroughly investigate your options. Visit potential sites and talk with friends and relatives about their experiences in their birthplaces. The more information you gather, the more informed will be your choice. In the following chapters, checklists will help you formulate your questions for hospitals, birth centers, and home birth practices so you can make the best decision for yourself and your family.

Some women will always feel safer in a hospital, and so that's where they should be. Others prefer to avoid the possibility of needing to be transferred to the hospital while in labor, although that happens infrequently. Still other women don't have adequate help at home to make an early discharge safe. Finally, epidurals and other types of regional anesthesia are only available in hospitals.

On the other hand, some women are comfortable only at home. They feel that in any other setting they are still on someone else's "turf" rather than on their own and so have less control over their experience.

Keep in mind that in any setting, safety doesn't depend on your actual physical environment as much as *who* is there and *how* the birth takes place. As one midwife told us, "Good midwives guard your birth experience, wherever they are working, whether it is in a hospital ward or the privacy of your home."

6

Hospitals

One of the nice things about nurse-midwives is that they provide options in birthplace choices. In this chapter we discuss the advantages and disadvantages of a hospital birth and consider how your midwife can help you have a positive experience in this setting.

Why Choose a Hospital Birth?

Hospitals remain the most popular birthplace choice of women today. Many women choose a hospital birth simply because it's the most acceptable choice in our society and don't even consider alternatives. But there are distinct advantages and disadvantages to giving birth in a hospital that are worth consideration.

There is no doubt that the biggest advantage of giving birth in a hospital is its emergency care, with on-site physicians, anesthesia, and operating rooms. Some women choose hospital birth because they want to have the option of an epidural, which isn't available in other settings. Others favor the hospital as a place to get a reprieve from family demands, or as one mother of three said, "I want my two days in bed with meals brought to me on a tray, because it's the only break I'll have once the new baby arrives."

Also, some women prefer to give birth in a hospital because they don't want to take the chance of being transferred to a hospital from home or a birth center if they develop a complication. When under the care of a midwife, an additional advantage of a hospital birth is that the client has a greater chance of continuing her care with a midwife if she develops a complication. Hospital-based CNMs typically have a wider scope of practice than they do in other settings, since physician consultation is readily available, as well as access to high tech equipment.

As one client told us, "I chose a hospital birth because my husband thought it was the safest place. I was lucky because my midwife stayed with me throughout labor. When there was a complication, the consulting physician arrived but allowed my midwife to continue taking care of me. She let me know she'd be standing by if needed. It was the best of both worlds for me."

But along with these advantages are some clear disadvantages. Some hospitals are very strict about what women in labor are allowed to do. The staff may not be as responsive to your needs as they would be in a birth center or at home. You may not be allowed to take a shower or a bath, eat, drink a glass of juice, or get into different positions. And some hospitals still require you to be hooked to an IV and fetal monitor, so walking around may be impossible. Some hospitals have started to relax these rules, but others haven't.

Also, the supposed "safety" of a hospital isn't always what it's reputed to be, as we discuss further on. Many women resent the intrusion into their privacy that is inevitable in a hospital as people they've never met wander in and out of their room taking blood or emptying the wastebasket. There is no doubt that when you give birth in a hospital you have a much higher chance of being exposed to medical technology. As one CNM said, "It is rare to see a normal birth occur in any kind of institutional setting. I mean *normal* as in no unnecessary intervention—to see labor unfold, to see it just happen the way it is supposed to happen for that individual woman." It is more likely that there will be institutional policies that you will have to follow even if you don't agree with them. You are less likely to be able to have your friends and family visit freely. Some women find it impossible to rest because of the frequent interruptions, and others don't want to be separated from their families.

Having a hospital birth with a midwife assures you of more input into how your birth takes place than with a traditional care provider. If you discuss your preferences with her in advance, you can expect to have a highly satisfying and family-centered birth a birth that includes your whole family—in the hospital.

Finding the Right Hospital for You

Many CNMs are authorized to use hospital facilities ("have privileges") at just one institution; others may be associated with more than one hospital, and you are given your choice. There may be more than one midwifery practice in your community with different practices working out of different hospitals. But even if only one hospital is available to you, you will want to investigate what it is like ahead of time.

Too often people assume that hospitals are all the same; in fact, they are not all created equal. Some are profit-making corporations, whereas others may be run by cities, churches, or universities. Depending on where you live, you may have access to anything from a large urban university teaching hospital to a small community hospital staffed by a small number of private physicians or, in some cases, only one physician. Each hospital has its own policies and standards.

A teaching hospital is usually the best equipped in terms of available technology and highly trained specialists. Therefore, it is probably the best place for you if you encounter an unusual complication in your pregnancy. It is also likely to offer the most advanced newborn care in case your baby has a problem.

On the other hand, the staff at such a hospital may have a high-risk bias, finding it difficult to make the transition from complicated high-tech care to a normal birth. If you are healthy and low risk, this may or may not be the best place to have a family-centered, low tech birth. Sometimes these hospitals have a separate birthing area for low-risk women, ideal for a midwife-assisted birth.

In any teaching institution, no matter the size, you may be exposed to medical students and residents who would like to be involved in your care. Although these caregivers can be quite competent and caring, you may start to feel like a guinea pig. Discuss your feelings about this with your midwife and she'll help prevent intrusions on your privacy.

The advantage of smaller community hospitals is more personal treatment. These hospital can be less busy, so they have more time for you. But they also may not be as well prepared for an unusual complication. And, as we discuss shortly, some small hospitals may not be able to respond as quickly in an emergency situation.

When comparing hospital settings, your best bet is to discuss the features of each with your midwife. She will know the characteristics and idiosyncrasies of the hospitals in which she practices. Also, procedures that are routine, such as requiring an IV or fetal monitor, in a certain hospital can sometimes be waived when you are under the care of your midwife.

It's a good idea for you to tour the hospital ahead of time so you can see what the birth rooms and postpartum area look like.

You will be less intimidated arriving in labor at a place that is at least somewhat familiar. If you have the chance to meet some of the nursing staff, be sure to ask them any questions you have.

Very few hospitals still offer old-fashioned delivery rooms. Most have updated their labor rooms so that they look more inviting, often with wallpaper, overstuffed chairs, and pictures on the walls. They still have medical equipment such as oxygen and blood pressure machines and fetal monitors, but the sterile-looking hospital beds have been replaced by birthing beds, which can be adjusted into different positions for labor and delivery.

Some hospitals call these rooms birth rooms or birthing suites or sometimes even birth centers, but they should not be confused with freestanding birth centers (see Chapter 7). Some hospitals have what they call an LDR, which stands for Labor Room, Delivery Room, and Recovery Room all in one. A few progressive hospitals have LDRPs (P for "Postpartum"), meaning you stay in the same room for the duration of your hospital stay. This is the best scenario, because it can be both physically and emotionally uncomfortable to move to another room during labor or just after birth.

As you investigate the physical layout of the hospital, remember that a pretty room doesn't always necessarily mean liberal, family-centered policies. The ideal hospital provides access to the latest in modern medical technology yet promotes family-centered and noninterventionist birth experiences. If you find a hospital that provides both ends of the birth spectrum, you'll also probably find a CNM practicing there.

A Sampling of Hospital-Based Midwifery Care

When we spoke with pediatrician T. Berry Brazelton, he discussed the CNM-staffed Midwifery Practice at Brigham and Women's Hospital in Boston, which is part of Harvard University's medical program. (The Midwifery Practice is connected with the standard Obstetrics Department at Brigham and Women's Hospital, but they maintain separate statistics.) According to Brazelton:

> The staff of nurse-midwives do most of the normal deliveries at Brigham and Women's Hospital. The program is working extremely well. Not only are the CNMs more compassionate, but they take, or should I say make, more time to work with the kids [siblings] and the parents. I think this family-centered approach to birth is here to stay, and I think it ought to be. I don't have anything but very positive feelings about the whole program.

Another CNM-staffed hospital on a smaller scale is in Cooperstown, New York. The Imogene Bassett Hospital is a small community-based teaching hospital that serves a large rural area as well as the town of Cooperstown. The first CNM came to Cooperstown in 1986 when the residency program in obstetrics and gynecology folded because of a lack of patients. Since then patients have flocked to the hospital, and now the staff of seven CNMs and three physicians performs 700 births a year.

Everyone at the Cooperstown hospital is an employee, including the physicians, so there is no competition for patients. All pregnant women are automatically cared for by the midwives, and those who are high risk are co-managed by a midwife and a physician. The chief of the obstetrics department, Dr. Mark Heller, said that midwives are "experts far in excess of most physicians when it comes to normal pregnancies." He noted that since the midwives joined the staff, the Cesarean section rate has dropped from 27 percent to 13 percent. The physicians do only surgeries and high-risk management, which is what they are best trained to do.

Cooperstown uses LDRPs, and women in labor are free to walk around, eat and drink, squat, and do whatever feels comfortable. Clients range from the very wealthy to those on medical assistance, and some travel great distances to get to Bassett rather than go to their local hospitals.

A hospital-based program that meets the needs of high-risk, low-income residents is the North Central Bronx Hospital in New York City. The obstetrics department is staffed by 29 full-time CNMs who provide care to all patients. This inner-city hospital admits anyone who comes to its door, and 70 percent of the patients can be classified as high risk. According to Charlotte Pixie Elsberry, Director of the Division of Midwifery, Department of Obstetrics/Gynecology, even though North Central has such a large high-risk population, this hospital has one of the lowest Cesarean section rates of all hospitals in the state of New York. Special care requirements for newborns and complications after birth are also far fewer here than in other hospitals.

Are Hospitals the Safest Place?

In our culture, most people still think hospitals are the safest place to have a baby. It is true that most hospitals have facilities that are not available in other settings. In an emergency, the operating room, anesthesia, physicians, and other trained personnel are at hand. For the few, very rare complications of labor that can be life threatening, the time it takes to get to a hospital can be critical.

On the other hand, the vast majority of births don't require this kind of specialized care. And a few characteristics of hospitals can actually increase risk. For example, since hospitals care for sick people, there is a higher chance than in a birth center or home birth that you or your baby will be exposed to infection. And, as we've said, you're more likely to undergo medical intervention in a hospital, which increases the risk to you and your baby of unnecessary procedures that can be more harmful than helpful.

As we've also said, hospitals vary greatly. Many are staffed around the clock by specialists, but a few small hospitals don't even have a physician on staff during odd hours (and that's when most babies seem to come), let alone a specialist. If you need an emergency Cesarean, you may have to wait for the anesthesiologist and obstetrician to be called in, which in some cases can take longer than the time it takes to come into the hospital with an emergency from home or from a birth center. In other words, the fact that you're in a hospital doesn't necessarily guarantee the fastest, most skilled care.

As a midwife who has practiced in all settings, Elizabeth feels lucky in the hospital where she's had privileges:

> The hospital is small and low key, and I can let women do just about anything they can do in the birth center. There's a shower they can enjoy, and they're free to walk the halls as much as they'd like. I can give them fruit juices to drink. And no one is watching over my shoulder. To me, the pretty wallpaper is less important than the way birth is viewed in the setting. In this hospital it's viewed as a normal thing.

Questions to Ask When Choosing a Hospital

Consider the following checklist of questions as you look for the best hospital for your birth. Discuss these questions with your midwife and with the hospital staff, if at all possible. Keep in mind that your midwife may be able to work around some of the hospital's routine policies. Also look for rating surveys that have been taken on hospitals in your area by newspapers, magazines, or insurance companies. Don't take these survey results too literally since sometimes higher Cesarean section rates can be the result of excessive referrals for complicated cases. The book *Women's Health Alert, Massachusetts* by Sidney Wolfe, M.D., Rhoda Dankin Jones, and the Public Citizen Health Research

Group (Addison-Wesley, 1990), lists the Cesarean section rates of over 2,000 hospitals across the United States. Such information may provide a gauge as to the amount of intervention used in a particular hospital.

If you plan to use a birth center or have a home birth, you can employ the same kind of checklist when choosing a back-up hospital in case of complications.

1. *What happens in an emergency?* Is an anesthesiologist available around the clock? If not, how long will it take to get into the operating room if I need a Cesarean?

2. *What are the admission procedures?* Will I be examined by someone else other than my midwife? Will I be hooked to an electronic fetal monitor, shaved, or given an enema?

3. *Are there medical students or residents on staff?* Will they be involved in my care?

4. *Will my activity during labor be restricted?* Do I have to be hooked up to an IV or monitors? Is there a shower I can use while in labor? Can I walk around while in labor? Will food and liquids be restricted?

5. *What type of newborn nursery do you have?* (Hospital nurseries are classified levels 1, 2, and 3. Level 3 is the highest classification, staffed by a neonatologist who can handle very sick babies who need to be on ventilators or require surgery. If you give birth in a facility with a level 1 or 2 nursery, your baby may have to be transferred to another hospital to get proper care if there is a serious problem.)

6. *Where will I be for labor and birth?* Are there separate labor and delivery rooms, so that I have to labor in one room and then move down the hall to deliver? Or will I be

able to stay in one room for the entire labor and birth? Will I be moved to another room after the baby is born? (Most women in labor want privacy, and being moved during pushing is uncomfortable, to say the least.)

7. **Do you have birthing rooms?** If so, how many are there? What is the difference between this room and other areas of the labor unit? Is the room readily available? Is it used frequently? Is there a waiting list? (Some hospitals have only one or two birthing rooms, offered on a first come, first served basis.) Are there restrictions on who is allowed to use the rooms? If so, what are they? (Some hospitals restrict the use of pitocin, anesthesia, or forceps in their birthing rooms.)

8. **What is the hospital's policy regarding my baby?** Is the baby sent to a nursery after the birth? If so, how soon? Can my partner accompany the baby to the nursery and watch the exam? Will my baby be fed supplemental bottles of water or formula? (That practice can complicate your attempts to initiate breast-feeding.) Is there rooming in? (Rooming in, or having your baby with you 24 hours a day in your room instead of in a nursery is highly recommended. This is the best way to get started with breast-feeding, so you can feed on demand or by the baby's schedule of eating rather than by the hospital's. In addition, you will be able to practice changing diapers and bathing your baby, as well as rocking and cuddling to your heart's content.)

9. **How long will I be required to stay in the hospital?** Do I have to stay a certain length of time, or can I go home when my midwife and I decide I'm ready? Will my baby be discharged early if I request it? (The baby's discharge time is usually ordered by the pediatrician.)

10. *What are the costs for the hospital stay?* (Costs are normally broken down by what supplies and facilities are used and how long you stay. It doesn't hurt to compare costs among hospitals. Find out what your insurance covers before you give birth. Your midwife's fee will be a separate bill and will probably be lower than a physician's fee.)

11. *Who can be with me during labor and birth?* Are there any restrictions? Can siblings visit? How about grandparents or friends? Can my partner stay overnight in the room too?

12. *If I have a problem that cannot be safely handled here, where would I be sent?* (If you live in a very rural area, the hospital may not be equipped to handle certain complications of pregnancy and birth. You would usually be transferred to the closest hospital that is better equipped, preferably with a perinatologist on staff.)

As you can see from this chapter, there is a lot to consider when choosing a hospital birth. Whether you give birth in a hospital by choice or by necessity, you should be able to have a positive and family-centered experience with your nurse-midwife.

7

Birth Centers

Although they're a relatively recent phenomenon, birth centers just may be the wave of the future. According to Kitty Ernst, founder of the National Association of Childbearing Centers, birth centers are "designed to build a woman's confidence in the design of her body and her inherent abilities to give birth and nurture her child." In this chapter we tell you all about birth centers and what it is like to experience a birth center birth with a nurse-midwife.

What Is a Birth Center?

Almost everyone has visited a hospital from time to time, but birth centers are a novelty to most of us. A birth center is a place for women with low-risk pregnancies to give birth outside a hospital.

101

It may be housed in anything from a Victorian house to a modern office building. It is typically furnished to be comfortable, with homelike birth rooms containing double beds, a family room with a kitchen so a family can gather to eat, and bathrooms with showers and often spas. As one woman who used a birth center described it, "The birth center was such a pleasant place to visit, I felt as though we were borrowing someone's home for our birth."

Birth centers are a hybrid of home and hospital. They offer the pleasant atmosphere of home, yet have medical equipment on hand and are normally located close to a back-up hospital. Catherine chose a birth center, although she really wanted a home birth:

> I chose a birth center even though it was an hour away from my home; it was located just two blocks from an excellent back-up hospital with a pediatric intensive care unit in case of an emergency. The hospital only five minutes from my home had very conservative policies and no pediatric facilities and would have been totally unreceptive if I had an emergency at a home birth and needed its facilities.

Some birth centers are owned by a group of midwives, physicians, or both, who are in practice together. Others are available to a variety of care providers, in which case several different practices may attend births there. Usually the birth center includes an office area for prenatal and well-woman care; in other cases it is just a facility for birth, with a different location for prenatal care.

Birth centers are usually licensed by the state in which they are located. Some have voluntarily undergone a rigorous process of accreditation by the Commission for the Accreditation of Childbearing Centers, which evaluates birth centers for safety and quality of care.

When we discuss birth centers in this chapter, we are referring to freestanding birth centers, or birth centers that are administered autonomously and are physically separate from a hospital. Although some freestanding birth centers are affiliated with hospitals, some hospitals use the term "birth center" misleadingly. Make sure your choice is really a birth center—where the midwife philosophy is adhered to, treating birth as a natural process—and not just a fancy name given to an updated labor and delivery unit.

History of birth centers

Birth centers evolved in the early 1970s in tandem with the feminist self-health-care movement. Using *Our Bodies Ourselves* (Boston Women's Health Collective, updated 1992, Simon & Schuster) as their bible, women were learning about their bodies and started questioning their health-care providers. CNMs became more popular during this time, since the two philosophies intertwined. Birth centers, in turn, created places that were more responsive to these women's needs.

As birth becomes more accepted in our culture as a normal, healthy experience and the economic realities of our health-care system are realized, expensive hospitals will likely be used less for birth and reserved for women with high-risk pregnancies who really need them. As one pediatrician told us, "Having a baby is a healthy experience that doesn't have to happen in a hospital for most women. Birth with a midwife at a birth center starts the baby off with an excellent foundation, providing better bonding opportunities between parents and baby."

One of the first freestanding birth centers, the Childbearing Center in New York City, was started in 1975 by the Maternity Center Association to provide an alternative for parents who were turning in frustration to unattended home births. Since then, birth centers have been developed in approximately 39 states, and as of this writing there are approximately 125 in existence, with another 60 under development. (See Appendix 2 for the address of the National Association of Childbearing Centers, which will assist you in finding a birth center in your area.)

Who Can Use a Birth Center?

Your midwife will carefully screen you for risk factors before you use a birth center, as we discussed in Chapter 2. Each care provider and individual birth center has its own screening criteria; whereas one birth center may prohibit a client who has undergone a previous Cesarean section from using the center, another will welcome her as they would any other pregnant woman.

Even if your midwife finds you eligible for midwifery care, she may not necessarily feel it is safe for you to give birth at the birth center. For example, if you have a breech baby or twins or go into labor too early—before 37 weeks—or too late—after 42 weeks—you will be "risked out" of a birth center to a hospital birth. However, your midwife may still be able to be your care provider in the hospital, or at least be there for labor support. Be sure to consult with your midwife about the birth center's admission criteria.

What Is a Birth Center Like?

Birth centers are designed to encourage individualized and family-centered care, active participation in the birth experience, and constant support in labor. There are few if any restrictions on you while you are in labor. You will be encouraged to walk around, drink, eat, lounge in the spa, take a shower or bath, or even go outside and stroll around the block.

Your family and friends are welcome. IVs and monitors are seldom used. Your labor and the baby's condition are monitored carefully, but in a way that doesn't interfere with your ability to do what's most comfortable for you. Rather than being strapped to a monitor and confined to bed, your midwife will periodically listen to the baby's heartbeat, wherever you happen to be, and sit by your side to assess the quality of your contractions.

Although pain medication is usually available, it is used infrequently in birth centers. Birth center staffs attribute this to the high motivation of their clients to give birth without medication, in addition to the greater sense of privacy and relaxation women feel in this setting and the center's ability to use other comfort measures.

The birth may take place on the bed, on a birthing stool, or wherever a woman feels most comfortable. There is no separate nursery to take your baby to—he or she stays with you, and all procedures and exams are done in front of you.

Birth centers are outpatient settings, and you are discharged between 4 and 24 hours after the birth, depending on how you and your baby are doing. You will be carefully monitored, and your midwife will decide when both you and your baby are ready to go home. Your midwife or the birth center nurse will keep track of your progress at home by regular phone calls and/or home visits. You will be taught how to monitor your bleeding, pulse, and temperature and to watch your baby's color and breathing at home. This will enhance your confidence in yourself as a parent, but will also let you know you're not completely on your own. After Catherine's birth,

> when we were feeling ready to leave the birth center, Elizabeth sat down and explained in detail everything my husband and I needed to know to take good care of ourselves at home. If we didn't remember something she told us (after losing all that sleep) it was comforting to know she was only a phone call away. It was especially reassuring to know a nurse from the birth center would be coming to our home in a few days to check on us.

A Sampling of Birth Centers

Although birth centers vary greatly in how they're owned, operated, and staffed, the following descriptions of two actual birth centers will help you get an idea of what you might encounter.

The Birth Place is a freestanding, nonprofit birth center located in the San Francisco, California, Bay Area. It looks pretty much like the other ranch-style houses in this residential neighborhood. Even on the inside, it is hard to discern that this is a birth center.

The well-appointed birth center has two bedrooms, each with a private bath and spa. There are a full kitchen and family room. While the Birth Place has a very warm, homey feeling, it has on hand plenty of emergency medical supplies, such as oxygen and suction equipment, tucked away in the linen closet. It is also located just ten minutes from Stanford University Hospital.

The Birth Place is used by a variety of professionals who have admitting privileges at Stanford University Hospital. A client can choose their care provider from among one CNM, one obstetrician, and two family practitioners. Doulas and nurses also help the birth attendants. Only the birth takes place at the Birth Place. Prenatal, postnatal, and well-woman visits occur at the individual provider's office. If a woman has to be transferred to the hospital for a complication, this birth center lets her return to recuperate in most cases.

There are strict requirements for clients who use the Birth Place. You cannot have had a previous Cesarean section or currently have a multiple or breech pregnancy, and pain medication is prohibited, no matter which care provider you choose. A woman can, however, give birth submerged in the spa, which is not allowed by many other birth centers.

There have been over 1,000 births at this birth center in the 14 years it's been operating. Of those clients, only 5 percent have required a Cesarean section, and less than 15 percent have needed to be transferred to the hospital.

Although the Birth Place caters to an upper-income clientele, the cost is less than a hospital birth, as explained later in this chapter under "How Much Does it Cost?"

Not all birth centers are used by upper-income women. Most are designed to meet the needs of women from all walks of life in the community surrounding the birth center. And a few have been created specifically to meet the needs of low-income women.

One of the first birth centers in the United States was created in 1972 to serve a clientele of Mexican-American migrant farm laborers who live below the poverty level. Their needs were not being met by the hospital over 25 miles away. Sister Angela Murdaugh, CNM, was the major force behind opening Su Clinica and then founding the Holy Family Services Birth Center in Weslaco, Texas, in 1983.

Holy Family Services Birth Center is comprised of six duplex birth units. Each unit has a family room, kitchen, full bath, and bedroom for birthing. The architecture looks much like the apartment complexes in the area.

Staffed by two CNMs, the birth center has a consulting obstetrician and pediatrician. The clients would normally be classified as having high-risk pregnancies because of poor nutrition, lack of family support systems, and other factors related to low income. Yet the birth center has been successful in keeping the pregnancies low risk through on-site nutritional counseling plus guaranteed transportation to the center so the women don't miss out on prenatal care. According to Sister Angela, Holy Family Services Birth Center has "half the rate of premature and low birth weight babies found in other hospitals in the state of Texas."

The center has a staff member whose sole job is to help clients obtain Medicaid benefits. The birth, along with the prenatal classes and counseling, normally costs about $1,000. If clients can't get medical coverage, the staff will work out some in-kind arrangement for payment, such as the client performing cleaning or landscaping work.

As you can see from these two above examples, birth centers cater to clients who can be worlds apart in socioeconomic status, yet yield similar results: Women who have safe and satisfying birth experiences with little or no intervention.

Are Birth Centers Safe?

Birth centers screen each woman carefully to make sure she is a good candidate for an out-of-hospital birth. They are staffed by competent, trained professionals, usually nurse-midwives, who are capable of handling emergencies. They have basic emergency equipment on site and a carefully thought out system for consultation and referral if problems arise.

In the National Birth Center study that appeared in the *New England Journal of Medicine* in 1989, researchers studied close to 12,000 women admitted for labor and delivery to 84 freestanding birth centers. The study concluded that birth centers offer a safe and acceptable alternative to hospitals and that such care leads to relatively few Cesarean sections. The satisfaction rate was very high; 98.8 percent of the clients indicated they would recommend the center to friends. The study concluded that "few innovations in health service promise lower cost, greater availability and a high degree of satisfaction with a comparable degree of safety."

A birth center can also provide an environment as comfortable as your home. The atmosphere is usually relaxed with few rules to get in your way. Yet you feel secure that it is a safe environment, too.

We spoke with Jane Brody, personal health columnist of the *New York Times*, who told us,

> Very few women need the high tech specialty care that's being administered by ob/gyn specialists. And the high tech

environment of a hospital is frightening when all you're there to do is have a baby. Normal birth will more and more have to move to birth centers. For the average delivery, you need something less than a fancy hospital—although you need ties to a hospital—very close ties for those unforeseeable emergencies. In moving birth out of the hospital you'll automatically bring down the costs: not just in terms of direct hospital costs for maternity care; you'll also avoid having to amortize the cost of all that fancy equipment—like CT scans and MRIs—that maternity clients aren't using anyhow. You will also reduce expensive intervention in the delivery, which is also usually unnecessary.

What if I have a complication?

If a complication arises at a birth center, what happens next depends on the specific circumstances. Your midwife will carefully and quickly evaluate what is going on, and if the problem is not easily remedied, she will call the hospital and/or the consulting physician to arrange for a transfer. This way, there will be no delay in your receiving appropriate treatment once you arrive at the hospital.

In the National Birth Center Study cited earlier, the transfer rates from birth centers averaged about 15 percent, with the vast majority being nonemergencies. Although people sometimes envision transfers from birth centers to hospitals as dramatic emergencies with sirens wailing, that is very rarely the case. The reality is that most transfers are for "failure to progress" in labor and take place in a very relaxed, unhurried way. Usually there is much discussion between the midwife and the family before the decision is made to transfer, and when it's time to go, everyone piles into the family car and drives together to the hospital. There the hospital staff and consulting physician are ready and waiting. If your CNM is authorized to use the hospital facility, she may well be able to continue your care if all you need is pitocin. If you are being transferred for a more serious problem such as fetal distress, the physician will likely take over, but your midwife usually stays with you for support.

Sometimes a complication is better handled at the birth center than by transferring you to the hospital. For example, if the baby appears to be in distress close to birth, your midwife will expedite the delivery and resuscitate the baby if needed. Many birth centers have arrangements with pediatricians who will come to the center if requested to be on hand for the birth or to evaluate the baby afterward.

How Much Does It Cost?

In general, the cost of having a baby in a birth center is about one half to two thirds the cost of having a baby in a hospital. Most health insurance companies and HMOs cover these expenses, but you should check with your provider to be sure.

Birth centers cost less because they aren't hospitals. They are short-stay settings and aren't required to have on hand expensive equipment that you won't use. The equipment that is there is used only if there's a good reason. The staff is small, and as one birth center midwife said, "We don't drive Jaguars."

Expenses at a birth center may be all inclusive, meaning the prenatal check-ups, birth, and postpartum check are included in one lump fee. For example, the Reading Birth and Women's Center in Reading, Pennsylvania, charges $2,100, of which $1,100 is the provider fee and $1,000 the facility fee. Lab work, the required visit to the consulting physician, and prenatal classes are not included in this fee and are billed separately. In other birth centers, the care provider's fee is separate from the facility fee. The Birth Place in Menlo Park, California, for instance, charges $2,500 for the facility, and the provider fee runs about $2,000. A hospital birth in the same geographic area would run $3,500 for the hospital use alone, and the provider fee would add about $2,500. (*Note:* All costs will most likely change by the time you read this.)

The popularity of birth centers not only with consumers but also with insurance companies is rising in conjunction with the increasing use of outpatient facilities in other areas of health care. A recent study by the American Hospital Association showed that in 1990, of the total 22 million surgeries performed, 11 million were outpatient, in contrast to only 3 million of the total surgeries performed in 1980. Insurance companies are also beginning to realize they are less likely to be covering the expense of a Cesarean section, costly anesthesia, or unwarranted medical intervention in a birth center birth. It is clear that if even a small proportion of the women who are eligible for birth center care choose a birth center, billions of health-care dollars could be saved nationwide—and some of those dollars could be yours.

Questions to Ask When Choosing a Birth Center

Most birth centers offer an open house or orientation session to describe their services and provide a tour of the building. If you are considering a birth center birth, you should take advantage of this service. Listed here are some questions you should ask the staff. In general, look for clean facilities and a warm and friendly but professional atmosphere.

If you have friends and family who haven't heard much about birth centers, bring them along for a visit. If they are misinformed and fear for your safety, usually a firsthand look will reassure them that your birth will be in clean and safe surroundings attended by qualified personnel.

1. *What happens in an emergency?* What hospital would I be transferred to, and how far away is it? Is there more than one back-up hospital I could use? (Use our hospital checklist on pages 97–99 to determine if the back-up hospital will also suit your needs.)

2. *In case of a transfer, do the midwives have admitting privileges, or will a physician have to admit me and manage my care?* If I transfer to a physician's care, will the midwife still stay with me? (We recommend you look for a birth center that allows your midwife to stay with you no matter what happens.)

3. *For what reasons would I need to be transferred?* What is the transfer rate at this birth center, and what are the most common reasons for transfers?

4. *What kinds of emergency equipment do you have on site?* (All birth centers should have oxygen, resuscitation equipment, emergency medications, and IVs readily available.)

5. *Who will attend my birth?* Will I meet them ahead of time? Although you have chosen a nurse-midwife as your caregiver, she will be assisted at the birth by other staff, usually registered nurses.

6. *How long has the birth center been operating?* Is it licensed by the state and/or accredited by the Commission for the Accreditation of Freestanding Birth Centers? (Accredited birth centers have met high standards for safety and quality of care.)

7. *Is there any medication for pain?* What other comfort measures are used?

8. ***Are there any restrictions on whom I can bring with me?*** Do children need their own support people? Is there a family room for visitors in case I don't want them to be with me in labor?

9. ***Do you have a spa, shower, or bath I can labor in?***

10. ***How long will I stay after giving birth?*** Is there a requirement that I stay a certain number of hours? If so, what is it?

11. ***What care do you provide after I've gone home with my baby?*** Will there be continued contact by phone or a home visit? When is my next office visit?

Having your baby at a birth center provides the best of both worlds. It provides the security of being close to a hospital, yet you feel at home and have the freedom to do what feels best while you labor. Birth centers provide the best alternative to hospital or home birth if either of those options aren't exactly compatible with your needs. But as we stated before, you should choose the birthplace in which you and your partner feel the most comfortable, since that will be the environment most conducive to a relaxed birth. Today, birth centers are growing in number across the country, and many experts believe birth centers will be *the* birthplace of the future.

8

Home Birth

Home birth is the third option for women and their families to consider when being cared for by a nurse-midwife. Since the turn of the century, when birth moved to hospitals, home birth has been given a bad name by the medical establishment and society alike. But we hope to turn that sentiment around. As we explain in this chapter, with careful planning and trained attendants home birth can be a safe and highly enjoyable experience.

What Happened to Home Birth?

Many of our parents and grandparents were born at home, and 80 percent of the world's population is still born at home. Yet home births in the United States have steadily declined over the years until they've virtually disappeared. The main reason for this decline is that our society has taught us to believe birth is a medical event best attended by a doctor in a hospital setting.

115

Even women who immigrate to the United States tend quickly to become indoctrinated in our cultural beliefs about birth, disregarding their own. According to Jennifer Dohrn, director of the Childbearing Center of Morris Heights in New York City, "Although birth centers and home births are more economically advantageous, many women from other countries feel they're 'in the United States now,' so even though they come from countries where midwives and home births are the norm, they want access to the hospital and expensive modern technology. We're working to change those attitudes here."

However, the last few decades have seen the start of a renewed interest in the home birth option. Some families are disgruntled with traditional hospital births and find that home is the only place in which they can regain control over how their birth takes place. Others just feel most comfortable in their own environment. The number of home births is still relatively small, and only a handful of health-care providers still offer this option in both urban and rural settings across the country. The majority of these providers are midwives.

Difficulties for the Home Birth Practice

Unfortunately, nurse-midwives who attend home births encounter some barriers that make their practice more difficult. Obstacles have been erected because of the stigma attached to home birth. For example, insurance companies are reluctant to give malpractice insurance coverage to home birth providers because they perceive home births as carrying an increased risk.

Besides the insurance problem, home births require increased responsibility for the CNM, travel time, more on-call time, and other inconveniences. Despite these constraints, the high degree of satisfaction both midwife and client derive from a home birth can make it all worthwhile. As Karen Laing, CNM, who has a home birth practice in Santa Cruz, California, said, "You really have to love women to have a home birth practice. You're giving women exactly what they want, and there's absolutely no substitute for a home birth."

Why the Home Birth Choice?

People may choose home birth for many different reasons. One of the most important reasons is that you have more autonomy over the birth than in any other setting. As one home birth client said, "In hospitals, the responsibility for something going wrong is usually someone else's, while at home it's mine." All decisions about the birth are made by you and your midwife—there are no rules imposed by any institution. This territorial switch can have quite a psychological impact on both the provider and the client because the client truly has a say in what goes on. In a hospital you're on someone else's turf, and you have to follow their rules and regulations whether they're supportive of your needs or not.

Privacy attracts many women to home birth. They view birth as a personal, private family event. Home provides quiet, undisturbed surroundings where everything is familiar and comfortable. As one home birth father told us, "When we visited the hospital they kept saying 'This is just like home.' If what you're trying to achieve in a hospital is a homelike atmosphere, why not just have your baby at home?"

Home birth is more convenient for you and your family. Your caregivers come to you rather than your having to travel during labor, which can be very uncomfortable. You and your family are usually most relaxed in these surroundings. You don't have to make special child-care arrangements, although a support person (other than your partner) for siblings is highly recommended. Sometimes a relative or a doula can serve this function.

Medical intervention is not readily available at home births and therefore is less likely to be used without good reason. This doesn't mean technology is not available at all, but it does mean that it won't be used unless it's truly needed. Karen Laing, a CNM, said, "We know women's bodies work! They can give birth, and babies are strong and able to come through labor and birth just fine. But health-care providers need to keep their hands off, leave them alone, and be patient in the process."

Many women prefer home birth because they're never separated from their newborn or the rest of their family, so there is a better atmosphere for bonding activities. Confidence in parenting skills comes more quickly since you have more responsibility for the care of your infant right away. As one home birth father told us, "One of the reasons we decided on a home birth was because we couldn't stand the idea of the baby being snatched away from us after birth."

The Cost of Home Birth

Home births usually cost less than birth center and hospital births, although that's rarely the motivation for home birth. For example, Harriet Palmer, CNM, who practices in the San Jose, California, area, charges $2,100 for a home birth, although the fee is negotiable depending on the family's financial and insurance situation.

In comparison, a hospital birth in the same location would cost $3,500 for the facility plus $2,500 for the provider fee. To further compare the home birth cost with a birth center, the facility fee at a birth center in the same locale is $2,500 plus $2,000 for the provider. The greatest saving lies in the fact that you're not subsidizing the cost of high tech equipment in the hospital. Also, you're not paying for the use of a birth center or hospital facility, so you avoid paying for their insurance, rent, utilities, and so on.

At a home birth you are paying only for the care provider and assistants and the minimal equipment needed to ensure safety.

According to Harriet Palmer, many private insurance companies cover home birth with a nurse-midwife. However, most HMOs will provide coverage only if you are using their approved provider or, in the case of Kaiser Permanente, their facility. Check with your individual insurance company to see if it provides coverage.

A Sampling of Home Birth Practices

The following two examples will help to give you a better idea of how home birth practices operate.

Family Birth Associates is a solo home birth practice in Alexandria, Virginia. Joyce Daniel, CNM, founded the practice in 1978 after being dissatisfied with hospital midwifery and realizing that risks were present with hospital births as well as with home births. She cares for about 25 women a year who live within a half-hour radius. Her clientele tends to be well-informed middle-class women who are screened carefully to be sure they are committed to the responsibility involved. All births are unmedicated, and the families are given a list of the equipment that is needed in addition to what the midwife brings. Joyce is assisted at the birth by registered nurses, who do a home visit at 37 weeks and stay for a few hours after the birth. Births are followed by home visits the first two days and office visits at two and six weeks postpartum. There are three consulting physicians, and Joyce characterizes the transfers as generally "orderly, calm, and predictable," usually for pokey labors or premature rupture of membranes without labor.

Joyce feels that people are entitled to safe options for birth. Her clients have other choices for nurse-midwifery care in hospitals and birth centers locally, but they are committed to having home births. Joyce finds this work fulfilling despite the long hours and responsibility. She said, "It feeds my soul."

Harriet Palmer also practices on her own, although she shares backup with two other midwives. They call themselves the Bay Area Midwives. In the past she had a partner, but now a lay midwife helps her when needed. Harriet has been attending home births for over 15 years and has helped at least 450 babies into the world.

Harriet has two physicians who act as consultants in case a hospital transfer becomes necessary. She is allowed to act only as labor support and not deliver the baby or provide other services when her client transfers to the hospital. Harriet said she doesn't have enough time to wait for hospitals to grant her admitting and treatment privileges since that could take 15 years or longer. She also finds getting malpractice insurance coverage an uphill battle and practices without it.

Harriet has two pages of strict screening criteria for clients; she says her clients "self-select" themselves in and out of her practice. "They eat well and take good care of themselves and make the best decision for themselves in taking care of their bodies."

Harriet has had great success with VBACs, or vaginal births after Cesarean sections. (VBACs are often prohibited from out of hospital settings even though recent studies support their safety.) She feels this success is due to the motivation of the mother, with the added benefit of her home being the right kind of relaxed environment for her second birth. She believes that many of the first Cesarean sections were unnecessary in the first place. Her transfer rate to hospitals is less than 10 percent, some of which occur during pregnancy because of twins or persistent breech and others during labor, usually because a little pitocin is needed to keep the progress of labor going.

Harriet said, "I don't understand why people have babies in hospitals to begin with! They give them all that 'fuss and feathers and whatnot' that they don't need. A lot of this technology has been proven over the years to not be needed for birth. It gets in the way of the woman doing the job herself."

Is It Safe to Have a Home Birth?

One home birth client put it best when she told us her philosophy: "You should give birth where you feel safe. Safety means being both physically safe and emotionally secure. I feel safest at home."

Most of society, the medical community, and certainly the insurance industry think home birth is risky. But the facts are that while unplanned and unattended home birth is indeed risky, a planned home birth following strict guidelines can be a safe undertaking.

Many studies have demonstrated the safety of planned home birth. And much of the unsafe reputation attached to home birth can be attributed to studies that did not differentiate between unplanned home birth and prepared home birth. There is a big difference between planned and unplanned home births in terms of safety. A 1984 study of home birth outcomes in England and Wales found the perinatal mortality rate for planned home deliveries was 4.1 per 1,000, whereas the rate for unplanned ones was a whopping 67.5 per 1,000.

The most comprehensive study comparing home births with hospital births was done by Lewis Mehl et al. in 1977 in northern California and reported in the *Journal of Reproductive Medicine*. The study matched 1,046 planned home birth women with 1,046 planned hospital birth women for maternal age, socioeconomic status, and risk factors. The births were analyzed for length of labor, complications of labor, neonatal outcomes, and procedures used. In the final analysis, home births had the best outcomes for both baby and mother. For instance, the hospital births had a five times higher incidence of maternal high blood pressure, three and a half times more meconium staining, three times more postpartum hemorrhages, and 8 percent more Cesarean sections. The infant death rates were essentially the same for the two groups, but three times as many hospital babies required resuscitation, and four times as many developed infections in comparison to babies born at home.

Obviously, a home birth can't compete with a hospital birth for access to emergency care. But as you can see from the Mehl study, there are several ways in which a home birth carries less risk than a hospital birth. One reason is that there is less risk for infection. You and your baby are exposed only to your midwife, her assistant, and your immediate family, and your baby is not put in a nursery. You also are less likely to be exposed to the unnecessary use of technology, drugs, and surgery, all of which carry inherent risks.

There is no doubt that in planning a home birth you are taking on additional responsibility. Since you will not have immediate emergency care available, it is essential that you plan carefully. In order to be safe, you must ensure that you are a motivated and healthy candidate, that you choose a provider who is a highly trained professional, such as a CNM, and that there is a well-equipped hospital nearby (preferably less than 30 minutes away) which will provide back-up emergency services if needed.

If you want a home birth, your CNM will screen you carefully to see if you meet the criteria. Guidelines for home birth are the strictest, and high-risk clients, such as those with high blood pressure, heart problems, or diabetes, are screened out. Each home birth practice has its own guidelines, and as in the other settings, your midwife will share these with you. Along with the medical criteria, she'll also be looking for psychosocial problems that may cause a problem down the road. She will want to be sure that you are committed to a home birth and are willing to take on the responsibility involved. You will also need to have a stable family situation with adequate support to help you after the birth.

Preparing for Home Birth

A home birth requires you to take full responsibility for your health and your baby's well-being. Because the birth will take place in your home, you need to be more involved in the preparation and provide some of the materials needed. Your CNM will inform you well in advance of the preparations you need to make. Most CNMs offer a kit you can buy containing everything you'll need at the birth, such as alcohol, sterile gauze, sanitary pads, and oil for massage. You may be responsible for the clean-up after the birth, although some home birth practices do this for you. To prevent staining, covering your bed and pillows with plastic is a good idea. (Some babies come out in a flash flood!)

Just as with a birth in a birth center, where you go home a few hours later, you also must take responsibility for your recovery care. You'll need plenty of help around the house for a week or so after the birth. If your family isn't available or willing, consider hiring a doula or a housekeeper for the first weeks, especially if you have other children. (See Appendix 2 for information on finding a doula.)

As with birth in any setting, follow-up care is essential for both you and the baby. Your CNM will advise you about how soon you should have a pediatrician check the baby. She will also inform you about her usual postpartum follow-up, which may consist of phone calls and home visits as well as a six-week checkup.

Questions to Ask When Choosing Home Birth

The following are questions to discuss carefully with your midwife before choosing a home birth.

1. **What happens in an emergency?** What hospital would I be transferred to, and how far away is it? Is there more

than one back-up hospital I could use? (See the hospital checklist on pages 97–99 to help choose a back-up hospital.) What is your relationship like with the staff? To be safest, the hospital should be within 30 minutes of your house, and it should be receptive to you and your midwife.

2. *In case of a transfer, do the midwives have admitting privileges at the hospital, or will a physician have to admit me and manage my care?* Will the midwife be able to stay with me through the labor and birth process if I transfer to the hospital?

3. *Who assists you at the birth, and what is her experience?* Most midwives who attend home births use birth assistants, who may be midwives, registered nurses, or other trained assistants.

4. *What emergency equipment will you bring?* Along with the doppler or fetoscope to listen to the baby's heartbeat and local anesthesia and suture to repair tears, the midwife should bring emergency medications, IV fluids, oxygen, and resuscitation equipment.

5. *What do I need to supply for the birth?* Will you make a home visit before the birth to ensure I'm prepared?

6. *How long do you stay with me after the birth?*

7. *How often do you keep in contact after the birth?* Will it be by phone, home visit, or office visit?

8. *How soon does my baby see a pediatrician?* What tests on the baby will be performed by you and when?

9. *How do I handle the neighbors?* Do they have to know I'm having a home birth?

10. *Who is responsible for the clean-up after the birth?*

Keeping Home Birth Available

Home birth is the endangered species of birthplace options. The difficulties in obtaining malpractice insurance, as well as the lack of willing physicians and hospitals to provide back-up services, are forcing some midwives to give up their practices. It is important that people realize they can make a difference in shifting attitudes about home birth. A planned home birth with careful backup arrangements attended by a qualified and experienced attendant can be safe. Consumers need to help educate their insurance companies, health care providers, and society at large if they want the home birth choice to be available in the future.

PART IV

Nurse-Midwife Specialties

Well-Woman Care and Minding Your Body

9

Not Just Birth:
Well-Woman Care
and Your Midwife

Most people associate midwives with birth, but your relationship with a midwife can form at just about any point in your life, from puberty through menopause, because all CNMs are educated to provide well-woman care as well as pregnancy and birth care. Many consumers don't realize that even if they never have a baby, they can still go to a nurse-midwife. Some CNMs restrict their care to pregnancy and birth, whereas others choose to specialize in the care of nonpregnant women; but most do both. In this chapter we explore the scope of the nurse-midwife's well-woman practice.

What Is Well-Woman Care?

Well-woman care refers primarily to women's gynecological health needs, which involves care of the reproductive system.

However, many women use their nurse-midwife as their primary care provider because they feel the most comfortable with her. In these cases, a woman may go to a midwife for her annual exam and Pap smear, but will not be seen by any other health-care provider as long as she remains healthy. A 1993 study sponsored by the Commonwealth Fund, which surveyed over 2,500 U.S. women, found that one third had not received basic preventive health services in the preceding year. Such studies give the nurse-midwife the added commitment to provide thorough health-care screening that goes beyond routine breast and pelvic examinations.

Well-woman care can include, but is not limited to, complete physical exams, initiation of family planning methods, care for specific problems such as common gynecological complaints, infections, sexually transmitted diseases, counseling on health habits, and on sexuality and menopause, and health screening for cancers.

Some CNMs, particularly those with additional training in family health care, can also manage the care of routine illnesses like colds and ear infections. Along with addressing these physical and medical conditions, CNMs are concerned about the psychological and social aspects of your health status.

As with the care of childbearing women and newborns, CNMs focus on the care of healthy women and work interdependently with other health-care professionals. They have the same collaborative arrangements with consulting physicians for clients with problems that go beyond the scope of their practice.

The Annual Checkup

As a midwife client, you may be pleasantly surprised to find the exam you undergo is often more detailed than the one you'd normally receive from a physician. Before the actual physical exam, your CNM will take your complete medical and psychological history. She'll ask you specific questions about your gynecological history, menstrual and sexual history, fertility history, and past use of contraception. She may inquire about your family and partner, your lifestyle, and your work situation.

The physical exam is comprehensive too. Along with the breast and pelvic exam, your nurse-midwife will usually check your eyes, ears, and thyroid, listen to your heart and lungs, palpate your abdomen, and check your reflexes. As she does the physical exam, she teaches you about your anatomy. If you are interested, she will give you a mirror to hold while she performs the pelvic exam so you can see different parts of your anatomy. She will reassure you about normal variations, such as one breast being bigger than the other or changes in vaginal secretions with your cycle. A lot of women, no matter what their education level, have concerns about their bodies and sometimes even harbor fears that there's something terribly wrong with them when, in fact, they're normal.

In her approach to well-woman care, Elizabeth explained, "I talk to my client as I do her exam, explaining what I'm checking and why. If I can tell she is ovulating by her cervical mucus, I tell her so. I find women are fascinated by this information, and it helps them to know their bodies better. Many women have mistaken normal changes for an infection and have worried unnecessarily."

The atmosphere is relaxed and unhurried, so you can ask all your questions without feeling as though you're taking up too much time. Catherine noted when she first switched to midwife care that she "always brought a list of my questions, a practice I'd gotten into from doctor visits. I soon found I didn't even look at my lists because the visit wasn't rushed. Plus, Elizabeth volunteered answers to questions that never occurred to me to ask."

CNMs are very adept at being gentle in their exams. They

are trained to be sensitive to women's responses and have learned by practicing pelvic exams on each other as part of their CNM training. From this hands-on approach, CNMs quickly learn what is uncomfortable for their clients! In the past, physicians learned by practicing pelvic exams on cadavers or on women under anesthesia. This provided no feedback about whether what they did was painful. (And male physicians in particular have no way of knowing what it feels like to undergo a pelvic exam.) Thankfully, many medical schools are now using paid, conscious clients for practicing internal exams.

Some women are particularly uneasy about their annual gynecological exam. Their anxiety may stem from a previous bad experience, such as a painfully rough pelvic exam or from having a history of sexual abuse. Also, women with nontraditional lifestyles, such as lesbians or single women who desire a pregnancy, may be concerned about judgmental treatment. These women often feel more comfortable with a CNM as their provider, since she tends to be more sensitive to their special concerns and supports individual choices.

Elizabeth had a client who during a routine exam, panicked when it was time for her pelvic.

> I immediately stopped, and we sat and talked about it. It eventually came out that she was harboring tremendous guilt over an abortion five years before. She came from a very strict family, and had never been able to tell anyone about the abortion. She no longer enjoyed sex, and it was taking a toll on her marriage. We agreed to defer the exam until she could work through her feelings, and I encouraged her to get counseling.

Many mothers choose to bring their teenage daughters to a CNM for their first breast and pelvic exam. They know their daughters will be treated respectfully and gently and will be educated about their bodies in the process. As one midwife said,

"My practice is naturally growing from my clients bringing in their daughters and their mothers for my care. One client told me she wanted her mother to have a Pap smear with me—she stopped having them because she was too uncomfortable with a male doctor."

Family Planning

CNMs have special training and are well informed about all methods of birth control. Your CNM will help you determine what is the best method for you only after first discussing your medical history, sexual relationship and habits, personal and religious feelings, and past experiences with different methods.

You and your midwife will discuss each method in detail, including how it works and its effectiveness, cost, possible side effects, and instructions for use. After this discussion, she will start you on the method you have agreed upon. She can prescribe the barrier methods such as the condom, diaphragm, cervical cap, contraceptive gels, foams, suppositories, and sponges or oral contraceptives such as the Pill or the long-acting hormonal contraception given by injection. She can insert an intrauterine device (IUD) or place contraceptive implants in the arm. She can instruct you in methods of "natural family planning" and counsel you about sterilization techniques.

Once you have started a method of contraception, your CNM will provide follow-up care. She will examine you periodically to ensure that the method continues to be appropriate for you and can help you to change if you have problems or decide you'd like to try something else. She will encourage your partner to be involved in this decision-making process as well.

Elizabeth was put in the position of marriage counselor when Catherine and her husband discussed vasectomy with her shortly after the birth of their second child:

I felt as though Elizabeth did a great job of staying impartial as we had this heated debate in front of her, although I secretly hoped she'd take my side. My husband was totally against vasectomy. He worried about the side effects. Elizabeth explained that vasectomy was a fairly easy procedure with a quick recovery. She discussed the fears that men often have about their virility and gave my husband names of other men who'd gone through it that he could talk to. She also provided pamphlets about the risks associated with it. I think we both felt we had the answer to our dilemma when she cautioned us not to go through with the vasectomy unless we were *both* 100 percent sure we wanted it.

Common Gynecological Problems

Most women experience a minor gynecological complaint at some point in their lives. Your CNM can treat you for such problems as menstrual cramps, irregular periods, vaginal or urinary tract infections, mild ovarian cysts, and premenstrual syndrome (PMS). She will ask you for a complete description of your symptoms and suggest nonmedical, holistic ways of dealing with the problem. For example, she may suggest exercises to cope with menstrual cramps or dietary changes to deal with PMS. She will teach you how to prevent the problem from recurring— for example, to drink lots of fluid and take vitamin C to prevent a bladder infection. Of course, in the case of extreme symptoms that don't respond to less interventive means, she can prescribe the standard medical treatment for problems. And in severe cases, the consulting physician is always available for consultation, collaboration, and/or referral.

Said one CNM client:

I'd had bladder infections for years before I went to my CNM. I was routinely prescribed antibiotics, and would end up with a yeast infection, requiring more medication. When my midwife heard this, she sat me down and taught me all that I could do to prevent these infections from happening. I followed her advice, and while I'm still prone to them, they happen much less frequently than before. I just needed someone to take the time to teach me how I could better take care of myself.

Health Screening and Prevention

At your annual visit, your CNM will screen you for other health problems and educate you about how to optimize your health status. She will perform or refer you for health-screening tests, including mammograms, Pap smears, colorectal cancer screens, and laboratory testing for cholesterol, diabetes, and other illnesses. She will question you about your eating habits, exercise, work, and environmental exposures and your use of cigarettes, alcohol, and recreational or prescribed drugs. Based on this information, she will counsel you about ways you can improve your health.

In her practice, Elizabeth finds that "for many women I see, this is the only encounter they have with a health-care professional. I tell them that I am obligated to discuss their overall health, so even if all they came for was a Pap smear, I am going to discuss how to quit smoking and get more exercise."

Your CNM will also explore your psychosocial background, including your relationships with your family and others, as well as your level of stress and the status of your mental health. These issues are of concern because your physical health can be very much influenced by your emotional health (see Chapter 10, "Minding Your Body," for further information). Since your CNM may have a close relationship with you, she is able to address personal issues such as battered woman syndrome or a need for family counseling.

The extent of counseling by nurse-midwives is best described by this CNM's account of a client in her urban practice:

> I asked my client in the teen pregnancy clinic how things were going. She said not too well. I saw a note in her chart about not getting along with the father of her baby. I asked, "Does your partner hit you?" The 13-year-old responded, "Yes, but only in my face." We talked further about this, and then I referred her to a support group for pregnant battered women that another midwife leads.

Sexuality

Most people in our society are not comfortable discussing sexuality, especially with their health-care providers. Many health-care providers are equally uncomfortable with the subject. However, sexuality is an important aspect of your health, and your nurse-midwife will take your sexual history as part of her information gathering. She will question you about your sexual activity, the age you had your first sexual experience, and the number of partners you have had. She will evaluate your risk for sexually transmitted diseases and counsel you about what constitutes safe sex as well as advise you on the best means of contraception.

She will also question you about your sexual satisfaction and any past or current problems with sex. Although many women hesitate to bring up the subject themselves, they usually feel relieved to be given the opportunity to discuss their concerns in a matter-of-fact way. Many CNMs are well informed about sexual issues and can be very helpful and reassuring.

Sexuality is often a particular concern for women at certain stages of their lives. Many have insecurities about their sexual feelings, or problems may arise at puberty, the first sexual encounter, pregnancy, postpartum, or around the time of menopause. Your CNM can help you anticipate normal events and changes that take place at these times in your life and advise you how best to deal with them.

One nurse-midwife told us:

> I find that while doing a teenager's first pelvic exam is a perfect time to bring up the subject of sex. Some teens come to me seeking birth control before their first sexual encounter and are happy to have someone tell them what to expect, and that the earth doesn't always move the first time. I also explore with them whether they're really ready for this step or whether they're feeling pressured by friends.

If you are experiencing problems in your sexual relationship, your nurse-midwife can offer you basic counseling, either individually or with your partner. If you need in-depth sexual therapy, she can refer you to a specialist.

Menopause

In recent years, CNMs have expanded their practices to include the care of older women. As clients grew out of the childbearing years and had new health concerns, they didn't want to give up the care of a nurse-midwife. Also, younger clients started bringing their own mothers in for exams, believing they would be more comfortable with a nurse-midwife. As the number of post-menopausal women in our society increases, there is an important place for the CNM's emphasis on maintaining health in aging rather than simply reacting to illness.

Much of the medical world views menopause as a pathological condition, signaling the end of life. Women are made to feel "used up" and not quite feminine anymore. These feelings that menopause is to be dreaded are compounded by our society's association of uselessness, senility, and death with aging.

Nurse-midwives promote a more positive view of aging as a

time for growth and wisdom. Menopause is viewed not as a disease to be treated but as a normal life event, similar in this way to pregnancy. It is a natural process that affects all aspects of a woman's life, not just her body. As in pregnancy, CNMs are uniquely prepared to help you deal with these life changes with support and compassion.

As one nurse-midwife client told us, "As I entered my forties, my periods began to get very irregular. I worried there was something wrong, and that I should see a doctor. My midwife was the only one who reassured me that these were normal changes that occur as you approach menopause rather than a dread disease."

Menopause is not a single event but rather a gradual transition that can begin as early as ten years prior to the end of menstruation. Your CNM will educate you about normal changes you can expect in your body and how to optimize your health. She will reassure you about common discomforts associated with these hormonal changes, such as hot flashes, vaginal dryness, and night sweats. If it becomes necessary, she can prescribe hormone replacement therapy, explaining both its benefits and disadvantages. But she will also advise you about natural ways to prevent or treat these symptoms through diet, exercise, and vitamin supplements. She will teach you about stress management and suggest you quit smoking, which can decrease these symptoms.

Like most CNMs, Elizabeth believes women should make their own choices, based on all available information. For example,

One of my clients was a well educated nurse. She was approaching 50, and her physician advised hormone replacement therapy. She had no problem with hot flashes or other annoying symptoms and really didn't want to take the medication. We talked at length about the apparent health benefits of the hormones, and she still felt it wasn't right for her. In some cases like this there's no clear right or wrong medically speaking, but she made an informed decision that I supported.

Your nurse-midwife will also discuss with you health concerns associated with aging, such as heart disease, osteoporosis, and cancer. She will advise you about preventive behaviors and refer you to other health professionals as needed.

Menopause and aging are not just medical events but have implications for a woman's psychological, social, and sexual life as well. You may experience changes in your family, marriage, and work life that influence your overall health. You may need reassurance that you still have sexual needs even though the childbearing years are past. Your nurse-midwife recognizes these concerns and takes them into consideration in providing your health care.

As you can see, midwives are not just for birth. They provide a wide array of services to you throughout the course of your life. It's nice to know that perhaps the midwife who comforted you through labor will be there when the only babies on your mind are your grandchildren.

✳ 10

Minding Your Body

Midwives have known for centuries what the medical community is just starting to accept: The mind and body are really one, working together to accomplish various tasks that keep the whole organism functioning. In this chapter we explore this holistic philosophy and how the midwife incorporates it into her care.

How the Mind/Body Connection Works

Stress and other emotional factors can have positive or adverse affects on the workings of the body, from halting contractions during labor to gearing your body up for an especially strenuous performance, such as pushing during labor. This mind/body interaction is an actual physical process that has been seen under the microscope by the discoverer of endor-phins (the body's own pain killers), Candace Pert, Ph.D. Dr. Pert, the former chief of the section on brain biochemistry at the National Institutes of Health, found a "psychosomatic communication network" at work in the body. In simple terms, she found peptides that carry messages of emotion to receptors throughout the body and the brain.

In his book *Healing and the Mind* (Bantam/Doubleday, 1993), Bill Moyers writes that over 60 percent of outpatient visits to primary-care doctors are related to stress or to prob-lems connected with the mind/body interaction. Yet traditional medicine has been slow to recognize the mind/body connec-tion. Many health-care providers still go along with the tradi-tional view that the body belongs to science and medicine, whereas the soul and mind are under religious/psychological control.

Therefore, medical care in the United States tends to focus on medical history and physical symptoms. Psychosocial factors, behaviors, and lifestyle, which can trigger illnesses, are too often ignored. Patients are treated in a mechanistic way, giving tech-nology more credibility than what the patient has to say about his or her condition. Moyers reports that only about half of U.S. medical schools are starting to incorporate courses about the mind/body connection and to teach physicians to communicate with clients better.

The Midwife Approach

One unique characteristic of nurse-midwifery care is its holistic and personalized approach of treating both mind and body. The CNM, through her nursing and midwifery background, is trained extensively in interpersonal communication, counseling, and education. These skills assist her in promoting your emotional health and in exploring how your health is affected by other issues in your life.

Your midwife is aware that your physical health can be influenced by your state of mind in both positive and negative ways. Specifically, she will help you to see the possible connection between a physical condition and other events or stresses in your life. CNMs believe if you feel confident, relaxed, and strong, you are more likely to have a healthy course and outcome.

If you experience a physical problem, your midwife doesn't immediately look to technology for the answer. While she will always carefully evaluate what is going on in your body from a medical point of view, she will also look at the bigger picture. Your nurse-midwife is concerned about your overall well-being, not just your physical condition. She provides care that besides meeting your physical needs also provides for your psychological, social, cultural, and family needs.

In additional to traditional medical treatments, nurse-midwives use a variety of healing and nurturing approaches. Your CNM may be skilled in the use of specific techniques like visualization and imagery, relaxation and meditation, and stress management. Some CNMs have advanced knowledge of massage therapy and other alternative treatments.

Nurse-midwifery care begins with a comprehensive evaluation of your psychosocial background. This information enables your CNM to provide personalized care that meets your individual needs. In addition, it allows her to identify potential risks, which ultimately can help her to prevent or minimize such problems as postpartum depression.

Your nurse-midwife is sensitive to the psychological implications of pregnancy and birth and is informed about other issues of concern to women. She will address these nonmedical aspects of your health as she takes care of you in pregnancy, birth, and well-woman visits.

Nurse-Midwifery Care and the Mind/Body Connection

Pregnancy

People frequently make light of women being overly emotional during pregnancy, yet in addition to hormonal influences, women face many legitimate emotional concerns during this time. To begin with, your CNM understands that whereas you may be thrilled to be pregnant, it is common to experience at least some degree of ambivalence. She will explore your feelings about the pregnancy in a nonjudgmental way and support you as you adjust to this major life change.

As your pregnancy progresses, your CNM will listen to your concerns about the effect of the pregnancy on your relationships, your self-image, and your work life. She will reassure you about normal mood swings, unpleasant dreams, fatigue, and work stress that can occur in pregnancy. Your nurse-midwife will discuss body-image issues during pregnancy, such as feeling unattractive or that you look like a blimp. She will listen to your fears regarding the health of the baby, the pain of labor, something going wrong at the birth, and becoming a parent. This psychological support contributes to a positive pregnancy and sets a good foundation for a satisfying birth experience.

As one CNM told us:

> Second-time mothers often worry more than first-time mothers. They think their luck has run out and that they can't possibly have another perfectly healthy baby like the first. They may hear someone relate a story about an unfortunate outcome and think it will happen to them. I tell them worry is normal, but most mothers and babies do just fine. If your worry is real, let's tackle it. If it's not, let's worry about something that is real, like pollution.

Many women are particularly susceptible to the influence

of their thoughts and feelings during pregnancy. Your nurse-midwife is sensitive to this and will try to create an environment in which you feel safe, secure, and confident.

Richard Jennings, CNM, teaches his nurse-midwifery students at the University of Pennsylvania the "uterine ear" theory. In emphasizing the importance of communication skills with pregnant women, he instructs his students not to "say anything to the woman that you don't want to happen." In other words, he counsels his clients in positive terms about how well their baby is growing and how smoothly their labor will go. He believes that if a midwife is careful to always speak honestly but positively, her client will in turn be positive and confident in herself.

Nurse-midwives encourage you to be actively involved in your own care, and they facilitate your participation in health decisions. This empowers you to feel in control and responsible for the maintenance of your health. Your CNM will convey her trust that you are strong and capable of growing a healthy baby. She knows that if you are self-confident you are more likely to have a good pregnancy.

Labor and birth

Your CNM will continue to attend to your psychological needs during labor and birth. As we discussed in Chapter 4, in most cases she will be a reassuring presence throughout labor, providing support to you and your family as needed.

Women who give birth attended by a CNM report a higher degree of satisfaction with this experience. They often report easier labor and a better overall birth experience because of the emotional support they received from their CNM. Traditional obstetrics does not promote continuous support during labor. In the worst instances, the woman and partner are left alone for the duration of the labor while a nurse watches a monitor at her desk. The physician then arrives when the baby is coming. Midwifery care during birth helps to reduce the level of anxiety, which can help in lowering the need for pain medication as well as in reducing medical interventions. CNMs reinforce their client's positive perception of how they perform in labor. They know confidence in the ability to give birth sets the stage for better family relationships.

In her essay in the book *Nurse-Midwifery in America* (a report of the American College of Nurse Midwives Foundation, edited by J. Rooks and J. Haas, 1986), Dr. Lucy Waletsky, a psychiatrist and obstetrician/gynecologist, writes, "Obstetricians often focus on their delivery of the baby, while midwives focus on helping the mother to deliver the baby. . . . Mothers who have a positive feeling about their role in delivering the baby are more mentally free to bond well to their baby and to begin a positive parenting experience with their partners."

As we pointed out in Chapter 5, it is important to be comfortable with your surroundings or you may run into difficulties in labor. For instance, many women just don't feel safe unless they give birth in a hospital. A CNM in a birth center practice described a case of environment anxiety: "We had parents-to-be, a physician and a nurse by profession, who had a dysfunctional labor. Labor would start at home, and when they'd reach the birth center, the labor would cease. This happened for a day and a half. When we transferred her to the hospital, she promptly gave birth. We finally figured this was the only place where they both felt safe."

On the other hand, all labor nurses can tell stories of women who arrive at the hospital in active labor and then everything stops. It often takes a while for them to become relaxed enough in the unfamiliar hospital environment for their labor to progress.

As we have said, some women feel more comfortable outside the hospital. One mother said, "I really wanted to have my baby in the birth center, but for some reason my labor wasn't going anywhere. Finally my midwife told me that we should begin to think about going to the hospital if things didn't change in an hour. Somehow that was all I needed. An hour later I was holding my baby!"

Your physical environment is not the only important factor for a relaxed labor; you must be comfortable with the people surrounding you as well. CNMs tell many stories of women whose labor doesn't progress because of the presence of a person or persons who makes them uncomfortable. Often when that person leaves the room the labor progresses nicely. A nurse-midwife at a birth center said:

> In our center, we don't restrict who can be present. But if a laboring woman feels too awkward asking her mother or extended family to leave for a while, I'll suggest that she let me be the "bad guy," and I'll do it. It can be the worst thing for a first-time mother in early labor to be surrounded by excited family members who love her deeply and "can't wait" for this baby to come—that's a great way to inhibit labor!

Your nurse-midwife will encourage you to think carefully about who is best to be with you in labor. There is no right or wrong person, despite society's pressures, which may make you feel that your husband *must* be there or that your children will be scarred for life if they are present. You are the only person who knows what will make you and your family most comfortable. For example, although most couples are happiest when the partner is involved, in some cases women (and men) do better if he's not present. Or perhaps your mother wants to come to the birth, but her love and concern for you are so strong that her anxiety will rub off on you. And although in some cases you may not want your child present because you will be too concerned about her seeing you in pain and become too inhibited to labor, in other cases you may all be happiest if you experience the birth as a family.

On the other hand, you may involuntarily hold off giving birth until a particular person arrives—often your husband, or sometimes a child, a friend, or a caregiver. Sometimes women wait until things are in order in their households, such as arrangements for the care of other children. We all hear stories of people waiting to die until they see a certain person—the same holds true for birth. As one client explained this phenomenon, "After a bad experience, I switched midpregnancy to a CNM practice. I really knew only one of the nurse-midwives from prenatal visits and a friend's birth. When I was in labor, it dragged on for hours, and I went through all the other CNMs one by one until that midwife's hours started. When I look back I know that I was waiting for her—because once she arrived, the baby did too."

If you are having a vaginal birth after a previous Cesarean section (called a VBAC), your nurse-midwife understands that you will need extra support and encouragement and may have difficulty at the same point in labor where you had the Cesarean last time. Or you may have subconscious fears because of a bad outcome experienced by a friend or family member. If you had a previous unpleasant birth experience, or sometimes an even seemingly unrelated life experience, you may have unresolved feelings that interfere with your ability to give birth. Your nurse-midwife should be attuned to these issues, and rather than interpret your lack of progress as a medical emergency, she can help you work through your feelings. Many, if not all, CNMs report instances in which this supportive care has helped women to avoid an operative delivery. Elizabeth had one such situation:

> I had a woman in labor with her fourth child—the pregnancy was unplanned, and it interrupted her plans to go back to school. She arrived at my birth center completely

dilated and we rushed around to get ready for a quick birth. The next thing I knew, it was several hours later and she had no urge to push. As we talked I realized that she didn't feel ready to have this baby—she hadn't worked through all her feelings yet. I sat with her and we talked about the changes this baby was going to make in her life. Her baby was doing fine so there was really no need to rush her. Finally she decided she was ready, and with one push the baby was there. I was glad I knew her well because otherwise it would have been natural to assume there was something wrong, when all she needed was time.

Postpartum

After birth, you can expect to experience some emotional changes. On top of the usual physical fatigue, you may experience mood swings as a result of dramatic hormonal shifts in the early postpartum period. At the same time, you will be coping with your feelings about the birth experience, becoming a mother, and changes in your relationship with your husband or partner. You may experience a brief episode of postpartum blues, in which you find yourself crying for no reason.

Your CNM can help you anticipate these emotional changes and support you through them. If necessary, she can help you to differentiate what's normal from a more serious problem like postpartum depression. Normal "baby blues" begins shortly after the birth and is shortlived. A more serious problem, often called postpartum depression, can set in. It lasts much longer than baby blues, and women are sometimes hospitalized because of its severity. No one has yet figured out what triggers this depression, and there is no scientific evidence that it is hormonal in origin. There may be a genetic predisposition to the condition, or sometimes it can be attributed to the lack of social and psychological support following delivery. Mothers of young children are frequently isolated and have to live up to social expectations of what normal motherhood must be. If a mother can be encouraged to talk over her feelings with someone nonjudgmental such as a midwife, chances are she will experience less severe symptoms and will have an early recovery.

One study pinpointed postpartum depression as occurring more frequently in women who have experienced high-risk pregnancies. A 1993 study by the Yale University Child Study Center and the Johns Hopkins School of Public Health found that women with high-risk pregnancies need to have more attention paid to their emotional health since they are at greater risk for postpartum depression and are more likely to be persistently anxious about the health of their children even when the babies are found to be normal at birth. Researchers found that these worries don't disappear but linger for many years, influencing the way a mother perceives her child and causing problems in the mother-child relationship. The study recommends that medical personnel try to alleviate unwarranted anxieties of high-risk pregnancy by talking more openly about concerns with the mother-to-be. This type of emotional support is standard practice for nurse-midwives.

Other than birth

Even when you are not experiencing the upheaval of pregnancy and birth, your CNM is attuned to your psychological well-being. She will investigate your emotional health and screen you for problems like depression, eating disorders, or physical abuse. She is informed about issues of concern to women, such as body image and self-esteem, and can provide support and counseling on these issues. As always, if you have a mental health problem that goes beyond the scope of her ability, she will refer you to a specialist in your community.

For example, it is common to experience irregular menstrual cycles as a result of stress or a life change. Furthermore, women who live together will often find their cycles change so their periods come at the same time. If you develop abnormal periods, your CNM will be sure to rule out a medical problem, but she will consider these kinds of reasons too.

Or a sexual problem may be caused by a physical condition, but may also be related to something else, like a problem in communication or dissatisfaction with your relationship.

Your CNM is especially likely to discover a nonphysical cause for problems of this nature because she makes a point of looking at your life as a whole. By identifying a nonmedical cause for a medical condition, you are more likely to be able to avoid unnecessary treatment and sometimes to resolve the situation more quickly and completely.

What your mind can't do

As much as we want the medical establishment to recognize the mind/body connection, at the same time we hate to see women blame themselves or their thoughts for any misfortune that occurs. For example, many women fear that if they become upset or angry while pregnant, it will hurt the baby. This is not much different from old wives' tales that say such things as "if you put your arms above your head, the cord will strangle the baby." Stress and emotions are a natural part of life. Your CNM will be most concerned about how *you* are handling the stress. The baby will be affected only if you stop taking care of yourself as a result. In fact, we know that some stress is healthy—the stress of labor enables the baby to cope better with life outside the womb.

If you have questions about how your mind and body work together, you should discuss them with your nurse-midwife. Be aware that statements such as "It's all in your mind" usually indicate the caregiver can't figure out what's really wrong with you.

It is very important to understand that this does *not* mean that you are to blame if you have a slow or difficult labor or some other health complication. While it is helpful to recognize the influence of your mind on your body, its significance should not be distorted so that you end up feeling responsible for something you can't control.

The Art of Midwifery

Nurse-midwifery has a strong foundation in medical science. But most midwives agree that science is only one part of the art of midwifery. The characteristics that differentiate midwifery from traditional medical care include the midwifery philosophy, which views you as a whole person with the ability and the right to be involved in your own health care; the repertoire of skills, in addition to technical and hand skills, that facilitate normal childbirth with minimal intervention; and the use of intuition or spirituality.

But one of your CNM's greatest skills is her ability and willingness to listen. Not only does she take the extra time needed, but she trusts that you know your body better than anyone else and listens to your impressions of what is going on. As one nurse-midwife explains, "When I am having difficulty ascertaining a situation, I ask the mother to tell me what she thinks; I always believe what she tells me unless it is proven incorrect."

This can be a refreshing experience, especially if you've sometimes been made to feel you are incapable of knowing your own body. Besides helping you feel more confident and involved, CNMs feel it helps them in preventing bad outcomes. As Elizabeth said, "If a pregnant woman calls me at 3 A.M. and tells me something isn't right, I never brush her off, no matter how tired I am. When you work with mothers long enough, you learn that they often sense a problem before it shows up clinically."

The nurse-midwife provides comprehensive care that you can find only in very exceptional medical environments. She can play an important role in getting you in touch with your mind and body, so you will be able to recognize if your medical problem is created or worsened by psychological difficulties. In her years of experience with Elizabeth as her care provider, Catherine has found that "a good nurse-midwife alleviates the worry you have about your problem by first educating you and then providing reassurance."

PART V

The Future of Nurse-Midwives

11

The Future of Certified Nurse-Midwives

The number of midwives in this country and Canada is steadily growing, as is the number of women seeking midwifery care. Nurse-midwifery care is safe, effective, low cost, and highly satisfying to consumers. CNMs improve access to care and in many cases improve outcomes for mothers and babies. For all these reasons, we predict that midwives will become the established providers of women's health care in the not so distant future.

Breaking Down the Barriers

Despite the proven benefits of nurse-midwifery in this country, nurse-midwives face many barriers. The greatest obstacle was identified in a 1985 survey by the American College of Nurse-Midwives Foundation as *ignorance*. Many people simply don't have a clue as to what a nurse-midwife is or does. Not only is the average citizen unaware, but so are many health-care professionals. Some women are told by their doctors to stay away from midwives because they're unsafe, when, in fact, their safety records match and often exceed those of physicians. A 1993 meta-analysis of current studies by the American Nurses Association comparing women whose births were assisted by CNMs with women whose births were attended by physicians found that babies delivered by midwives fared as well if not better than those delivered by physicians. One striking statistic was that the rate of premature babies among physician patients was 10 percent, whereas the CNM patients' premature baby rate was less than half that, or only 4.5 percent.

Some of the confusion about midwives is due to the existence of different types of midwives practicing across the United States (see Chapter 1). Many midwives support the development of a single standard for professional midwifery, which would include CNMs and "direct-entry" (or nonnurse) midwives. The Carnegie Foundation for the Advancement of Teaching been involved in these discussions, which are ongoing as of this writing. If some standardization results, consumers will then be assured of the experience and education their midwife possesses.

Another difficulty midwives face is obtaining hospital privileges, which enable a CNM to practice in a specific hospital. Although you'll find CNMs practicing in many hospitals across the nation, many have had to fight hard to gain access to hospital facilities. Some hospitals block CNMs from using their facilities or place unfair restrictions on them, such as requiring the CNM be an employee of a physician or requiring a doctor to be present at their births. "The hospital is frequently the battlefield where economic, power, and control issues between nurse-midwives and physicians are being fought," according to Helen Burst, CNM, director of the Nurse-Midwifery Program at Yale University.

Two other issues that affect the CNM's ability to practice are prescription-writing privileges and third party reimbursement or payment of fees by insurance companies. As of this writing, 33 states allow CNMs to write prescriptions, and CNMs are working hard in the remaining states to obtain this privilege. Although most private insurance companies and all government medical insurance plans cover nurse-midwifery services, only 24 states have mandated third party reimbursement, which means insurance companies have to pay for CNM services. (Your midwife can tell you if your state is one of these.) However, even when CNM services are covered by medical insurance, CNMs are frequently reimbursed at a lower rate than physicians for the same services. Most HMOs and large insurance plans do provide coverage, but some of the new "managed insurance" programs exclude CNMs. You will need to check with your insurance company to see what it covers. If it doesn't provide coverage, it may simply be because the carrier is ignorant about CNM care. Some families have been able to convince insurers to provide coverage by educating them about the cost effectiveness of such care.

The Malpractice Issue

As we've demonstrated repeatedly, CNMs have an excellent safety record. Their rate of being sued for malpractice is much lower than that of obstetricians. In an informal 1991 survey by the ACNM, 9 percent of CNMs said they had been sued in the last ten years. In comparison, a similar informal survey taken by the American College of Gynecologist/Obstetricians the same year found that 79.4 percent of obstetricians said they had been sued for malpractice in the last ten years. These surveys were not done scientifically and were not adjusted for length of time in practice. Nor were the responses checked for accuracy by either group. Still, there is a clear indication that midwives are sued less frequently. Despite the few lawsuits against CNMs, they still have difficulty obtaining malpractice insurance. Many CNMs have found coverage through the ACNM, although their carrier currently refuses to cover CNMs who perform home births. Some home birth CNMs have been able to obtain alternative insurance, but those who can't find coverage are forced to either give up their practice or put personal and family assets on the line.

Also, when insurance is available, the cost may be prohibitively expensive. In Washington, D.C., for example, a policy can cost as much as $13,500 a year. This may not be excessive by physicians' standards, but this amount constitutes a large portion of a typical CNM's income. Another problem is that insurance companies sometimes punish physicians who work with nurse-midwives, either by canceling their policies or by charging them more. In fact, the Federal Trade Commission had to intervene in a case, prohibiting such discrimination as an unfair trade practice, which makes it illegal.

The American Way

Our health-care system is under heavy criticism, particularly in the area of maternal/child health care. Jennifer Howse, Ph.D., president of the March of Dimes Birth Defect Foundation, told us:

> There is a general consensus that America must find ways to significantly improve birth outcomes. To do this, health-care reform must address critical issues in perinatal, or before and after childbirth, care for women. At a minimum, we need a dramatically increased emphasis and financial investment in prevention services, including early and better risk assessment and preconceptional care, and CNMs need to be part of the system.

The United States spends 14 percent of its gross domestic product on health care—more than any other nation—according to a 1990 report by the Organization for Economic Development and Cooperation. Yet the death rate for infants in the United States is 9.8 per 1,000 births, ranking it twenty-second among other industrialized nations, according to 1989 statistics from the Center for Disease Control. It's obvious we're all spending more for health care and getting less.

Poor women and women living in rural areas are particularly underserved by the U.S. health-care system. There is a shortage of providers to care for these women, who are in the most need.

Our priorities are out of kilter: Birth is viewed as an illness rather than a normal life event. As a result, we pour money into new technology rather than good prenatal and preventive care. Rather than spending health-care dollars on preventing preterm birth, we spend it on expensive machines to save the lives of the high-risk babies that result from poor prenatal care. Howse pointed out, "Every dollar we spend on good prenatal care saves us three dollars in medical costs."

Furthermore, medical intervention has become routine. The United States ranks third highest in the world for Cesarean sections, which are performed in 23 out of 100 births, according to a 1992 report by the American Medical Association. According to the April 1991 *Health Letter* published by the Public Citizen Health Research Group, half of these Cesarean sections are unnecessary and amount to billions of dollars in health-care costs.

Anthropologist Robbie Davis-Floyd told us:

The scary thing about birth today is that there's so much technology embedded in the process that machines threaten to take over the birth experience from the woman. The hope arises that technology will one day take a back seat in the birth process, bringing birth back to what it really is, a natural function that a woman's body is quite capable of achieving with emotional support and comfortable surroundings.

Midwives as the Solution

We hope for a future in which nurse-midwives, as the specialists in normal birth, will be the primary care providers for women. As gatekeepers, they will determine who requires specialized care, thereby reserving the physician's area of expertise for where it belongs—with high-risk, complicated cases.

Pediatrician T. Berry Brazelton agrees, stating, "I don't think M.D.s are doing everything for people that they wish they were. Because of this, I think we're in for a big change in the birth scene in the future. In all likelihood, CNMs will take over normal births, while physicians will take care of the high-risk maternity cases." Obstetrician/gynecologist Don Creevy added,

> The role of the obstetrician is changing. Increasingly he or she will be trained to manage high-risk pregnancies in cooperation with midwives and to back midwives as they attend low-risk births. Fewer obstetricians per capita will be needed in the future, because more births will be attended by midwives. For this to happen, there must be a major shift in the attitudes of obstetricians, family physicians, pediatricians, and hospital administrators toward nurse-midwives.

In some areas of the country, greater utilization of nurse-midwives is already being implemented. The state advisory to Florida's Healthy Start Program has recommended that the state work toward an objective of having 50 percent of normal pregnancies attended for by midwives by the year 2000.

In discussions of health-care reform, the nurse-midwifery profession comes up repeatedly because many of the proposed solutions to today's health-care crisis are already offered by midwifery. CNMs have been leaders in providing care in under-served areas of the country; in focusing on prevention, health education, and improving health behaviors; and in cost containment. In her proposal for the Clinton Task Force on Health Care, Catherine Carr, CNM, Ph.D. stated, "Cost savings associated with midwifery come from a reduction of the Cesarean section rate, judicious use of technology, and the reduction in poor outcomes, especially low birth weight babies, often associated with women who are high risk due to social circumstances or poor life style and health habits."

Realizing the cost savings when utilizing CNMs is plain to see. Not only are midwife fees usually about 30 percent to 40 percent less than those of physicians, but the direct cost associated with educating midwives is approximately one fourth to one fifth that for physicians, according to the Office of Technology Assessment. Also, salaries are worlds apart for the two professions. According to a 1991 survey by the American College of Gynecologists, average private obstetrician/gynecologists earn $198,380 after taxes. Nurse-midwives in comparison earn approximately less than one quarter of that, as reported in "The Findings of the 1991 Annual American College of Nurse-Midwives Membership Survey," published in the *Journal of Nurse Midwifery* (Vol. 38, no. 1).

Joyce Thompson, past president of the ACNM, asked:

> What will it cost *not* to invest in pregnancy as health, nurse-midwives and nurse-practitioners as the primary health partners with women and childbearing families. How much longer can society ignore the fact that women cared for by CNMs adopt healthier behaviors, have less preterm births, fewer low birth weight infants, and better parenting skills?

Obstetrician/gynecologist Don Creevy said:

> I believe one of the beneficial effects of President Clinton's health-care reform program will be the discovery

that CNMs are very cost effective care providers. They are able to work at a substantially lower hourly rate than physicians. With fewer routine interventions in the birth process by midwives will come not only better outcomes for mothers and babies but also substantially reduced costs.

Besides CNMs becoming the primary-care providers for normal births, we envision a future in which birth takes place primarily in freestanding centers, with hospitals being reserved for women who are truly in need of expensive technology. According to Kitty Ernst, director of the National Association of Childbearing Centers, "We need to educate the public that the whole system is upside down; healthy women shouldn't be admitted to acute care to give birth. We need to approach pregnancy and birth as normal until proven otherwise. This makes it logical for women to go to birth centers and be transferred to hospitals only if they need it."

The need for more CNMs

CNMs can certainly help remedy our health-care crisis but, unfortunately, there aren't enough of them to do it. Currently there are about 4,500 CNMs in the United States, and until recently, educational programs produced only a few hundred a year. The ACNM has taken on this challenge by stating that it hopes to produce 10,000 CNMs by the year 2001.

According to Ruth Lubic, CNM, director of the Maternity Center Association, "I think the reason we don't have more nurse-midwives at this point is that we've been kept small by the medical control of training sites. If the doctors on a hospital staff don't want to let students of nurse-midwifery in, the students don't get in."

CNMs are looking at new ways to recruit and train nurse-midwives. One example is the Community-Based Nurse-Midwifery Program, which is part of the Frontier Nursing Service.

Elizabeth is currently working with this educational program, which allows nurses to remain in their home community while pursuing their training—thus meeting two needs: providing a mechanism for nurses who cannot relocate to pursue graduate study and making available new CNMs to serve communities that lack such services. Since 1989, this program has graduated over 100 CNMs, and over 300 more students are currently enrolled. Several other programs are looking at incorporating distance learning technology into their curricula to expand the student base.

Back to the Future

In many respects we need to go back to the time when midwives were the primary care providers for birth. As more and more people learn about her role, the CNM will gain a secure place in the health care of this country.

CNMs are involved in many endeavors beyond caring for families, including education of future nurse-midwives and other health-care professionals such as medical students, residents, and student nurses; development of health policy on local and national levels; research in women's health care, with particular focus on the effectiveness of midwifery management; and promotion of better health for women worldwide, serving in Third World countries as educators, advisers, and providers.

If and when midwives become the routine caregivers for childbearing women, as is the case in many of the countries with infant mortality statistics superior to ours, then we will succeed in saving money as well as improving access and outcomes.

You can play a role in ensuring that all women have access to midwifery care. Support nurse-midwives individually on a local level and as a profession nationally and internationally. Support legislation proposed to ease the prejudicial burdens

CNMs face. Most important, talk to your friends and family about the safe and satisfying care that nurse-midwives provide.

A good example of how obstetricians might run their practices one day is exactly how Jane Brody told us her physician practices now: "My obstetrician/gynecologist has several CNMs that work with him. He takes pictures [for the parents] while the nurse-midwives attend the births!"

�֎ *Appendix 1*

Suggested Reading

We use the following books in our research and recommend them for further reading.

Birth: Philosophy/Cultural Influences

Davis-Floyd, Robbie. *Birth as an American Rite of Passage.* Berkeley: University of California Press, 1992.

Jordan, Brigette. *Birth in Four Cultures.* Prospect Heights, IL: Waveland Press, 1993.

Mitford, Jessica. *The American Way of Birth.* New York: E. P. Dutton, 1992.

Rothman, Barbara Katz. In *Labor: Women and Power in the Birthplace.* New York: W. W. Norton, 1991.

Well-Woman Care

Kitzinger, Sheila. *Woman's Experience of Sex*. New York: G. P. Putnam's, 1983.

Love, Susan, with Karen Lindsay. *Dr. Susan Love's Breast Book*. Reading, MA: Addison-Wesley, 1990.

The New Our Bodies Ourselves, A Book by and for Women. Boston Women's Health Book Collective. New York: Simon & Schuster, 1992.

Perry, Susan, and Kate O'Hanlan. *Natural Menopause*. Reading, MA: Addison-Wesley, 1992.

Wolfe, Sidney, M., M.D. *Women's Health Alert, Massachusetts*. Reading, MA: Addison-Wesley, 1990.

History of Midwifery

Breckenridge, Mary. *Wide Neighborhoods: A Story of the Frontier Nursing Service*. Lexington: University Press of Kentucky, 1981.

Ehrenreich, Barbara, and Deirdre English. *Witches, Midwives, and Nurses: A History of Women Healers*. Old Westbury, NY: The Feminist Press, SUNY, 1973.

Leavitt, Judith Walzer. *Brought to Bed: Childbearing in America 1750–1950*. New York: Oxford University Press, 1986.

Litoff, Judy Barrett. *The American Midwife Debate: A Sourcebook on Its Modern Origins*. New York: Greenwood Press, 1986.

Scholten, Catherine M. *Childbearing in American Society 1650–1850*. New York: New York University Press, 1985.

Ulrich, Laurel Thatcher. *A Midwife's Tale, The Life of Martha Ballard, Based on Her Diary, 1785–1812*. New York: Alfred A. Knopf, 1990.

Wertz and Wertz. *Lying-In: A History of Childbirth in America*. New Haven, CT: Yale University Press, 1989.

Midwifery

Armstrong, Penny, and Sheryl Feldman. *A Midwife's Story.* New York: Ballantine Books, 1986.

Logan, Onnie Lee, as told to Katherine Clark. *Motherwit, an Alabama Midwife's Story.* New York: E. P. Dutton, 1989.

Rooks, J., and J. Haas, eds. *Nurse-Midwifery in America: A Report of the ACNM Foundation.* Washington, DC: ACNM, 1986.

Pregnancy and Birth

American College of Nurse-Midwives and Sandra Jacobs. *Having Your Baby with a Nurse-Midwife.* New York: Hyperion Books, 1993.

Armstrong, Penny, and Sheryl Feldman. *A Wise Birth: Bringing Together the Best of Natural Childbirth with Modern Medicine.* New York: William Morrow, 1990.

Chalmers, Ian, Murray Enkin, and Marc Keirse. *A Guide to Effective Care in Pregnancy and Childbirth.* New York: Oxford University Press, 1989.

Kitzinger, Sheila. *The Complete Book of Pregnancy and Birth.* New York: Alfred A. Knopf, 1989.

Kitzinger, Sheila. *Your Baby, Your Way: Making Pregnancy Decisions and Birth Plans.* New York: Pantheon Books, 1987.

Klaus, Marshall, Kennel Klaus, and Phyllis Klaus. *Mothering the Mother.* Reading, MA: Addison-Wesley, 1993.

La Leche League International. *The Womanly Art of Breast-feeding.* Franklin Park, IL: 1991.

McCartney, Marion, and Antonia van der Meer. *The Midwife's Pregnancy and Childbirth Book: Having Your Baby Your Way.* New York: Henry Holt, 1990.

Child Development

Brazelton, T. Berry. *Touchpoints, the Essential Reference.* Reading, MA: Addison-Wesley, 1993.

Leach, Penelope. *Babyhood.* New York: Alfred A. Knopf, 1976.

Leach, Penelope. *Your Baby and Child: From Birth to Age Five.* New York: Alfred A. Knopf, 1990.

Mind and Body

Borysenko, Joan. *Minding the Body, Mending the Mind.* New York: Bantam Books, 1987.

Coleman, Dan, and Joel Gurn, eds. *Mind Body Medicine.* Yonkers, NY: Conumer Reports Books, 1993.

Cousins, Norman. *Head First.* New York: E. P. Dutton, 1989.

Moyers, Bill. *Healing and the Mind.* New York: Bantam/ Doubleday, 1993.

Peterson, Gayle, and Lewis Mehl. *Pregnancy as Healing.* Berkeley, CA: Mindbody Press, 1984.

Appendix 2

Organizations

U.S. and Canadian organizations are included here.

Doulas

National Association of Postpartum Care Services
326 Shields Street
San Francisco, CA 94132-2734

Midwifery

American College of Nurse-Midwives
818 Connecticut Avenue NW, Suite 900
Washington, DC 20006
(202) 728-9860
Fax (202) 728-9897

Midwives' Alliance of North America
   600 Fifth Street
   Monett, MO 65708

Childbirth Education

American Academy of Husband-Coached Childbirth (Bradley method)
   P.O. Box 5224
   Sherman Oaks, CA 91413
   (818) 788-6662

American Society for Psychoprophylaxis in Obstetrics (ASPO/Lamaze)
   1101 Connecticut Avenue N.W., Suite 700
   Washington, DC 20036
   (800) 368-4404
   This number can also refer Canadian callers to training programs and instructors in Canada.

International Childbirth Education Association
   P.O. Box 20048
   Minneapolis, MN 55420-0048
   (612) 854-8660
   Write the Canadian director care of this address.

Breast-feeding

LaLeche League International
   9616 Minneapolis Avenue
   Franklin Park, IL 60131
   (708) 455-7730

LaLeche League of Canada
   18C Industrial Drive, Box 29
   Chesterville, Ontario KOC1HO
   (613) 448-1842

Ligue La Leche
    Box 874
    Ville St. Laurent
    Quebec, Canada H4L4W3
    (514) 747-9127

Women's Health

Boston Women's Health Book Collective
    47 Nicholls Avenue
    Watertown, MA 02172
    (617) 924-2681

Coalition for the Medical Rights of Women
    1638-B Haight Street
    San Francisco, CA 94117

Feminist Women's Health Centers Federation
    6221 Wilshire Boulevard
    Los Angeles, CA 90048
    (213) 938-9838

Health Sharing, Inc.
    14 Skey Lane
    Toronto, Ontario N6J354
    (416) 532-0812
    Publishes magazine on women's health from a feminist
    perspective.

Lesbian Health Fund, American Association of Physicians for
Human Rights
    273 Church Street
    San Francisco, CA 94114

National Action Committee on the Status of Women
    Health Committee
    57 Mobile Drive
    Toronto, Ontario M4a 1HS
    (416) 759-5252

National Women's Health Network
    1325 G Street N.W., Lower Level
    Washington, DC 20005
    (202) 347-1140

Planned Parenthood Federation of America
    Call your local chapter.

Cesarean Birth

Cesarean Prevention Movement
    P.O. Box 152
    University Station
    Syracuse, NY 13210
    (315) 424-1942

C/SEC (Cesareans, Support Education & Concern)
    22 Forest
    Framingham, MA 01701
    (508) 877-8266

Birth Centers

Maternity Center Association
    48 E 92 Street
    New York, NY 10128
    (212) 369-7300

National Association of Childbearing Centers
    R.D. 1, Box 1
    Perkiomenville, PA 18074
    (215) 234-8068

Home Birth

Association for Childbirth at Home, International
P.O. Box 39498
Los Angeles, CA 90039
(213) 667-0839

Informed Homebirth
P.O. Box 3675
Ann Arbor, MI 48106
(313) 662-6857

Birth: General

American Foundation for Maternal Child Health
439 E 51 Street
New York, NY 10022
(212) 759-5510

March of Dimes
Birth Defect Foundation
Professional Education Department
1275 Mamaroneck Avenue
White Plains, NY 10605

National Association of Professionals for Safe Alternatives in
Childbirth (NASAC)
Route 1
Box 646
Marble Hill, MO 63764
(314) 238-2010

Appendix 3

Educational Programs

Certificate Programs

Baylor College of Medicine *97

Nurse-Midwifery Education Program
Dept. of OB/GYN
Smith Towers, 7th Floor
6550 Fannin
Houston, TX 77030
(713) 793-3541, 3542
Program Director:
Susan Wente, CNM, MPH

Baystate Medical Center†

Nurse-Midwifery Education Program
689 Chestnut Street
Springfield, MA 01199
(413) 784-4448
Program Director:
Susan DeJoy, CNM, MSN

Charles R. Drew University of Medicine & Science *97
  Nurse-Midwifery Education Program
  College of Allied Health Sciences
  1621 East 120th Street
  Los Angeles, CA 90059
  (213) 563-4951, 603-4611
  Program Director:
  Gwendolyn Spears, CNM, MSN
  (MSN option available from U of CA)

Education Program Associates
Midwifery Education Program *97
  1 West Campbell Avenue
  Campbell, CA 95008
  (408) 374-3720
  Program Director:
  Linda Walsh, CNM, MPH, PhD

Frontier School of Midwifery and Family Nursing *97
Community-Based Nurse-Midwifery Education Program
  PO Box 528
  Hyden, KY 41729
  (606) 672-2312
  Program Director:
  Mary Kate McHugh, CNM, MSN
  *(MSN and ND option available from Case Western
  University)*

Parkland School of Nurse-Midwifery *96
  Parkland Memorial Hospital
  In affiliation with Univ. of Texas
  SW Medical Center at Dallas
  5th Floor, WCS Department
  5201 Harry Hines Blvd.
  Dallas, TX 75235
  (214) 590-8597 or 8107
  Program Director:
  Mary C. Brucker, CNM, DNSc
  (MS option avail. from TX Women's Univ.)

State University of New York *98
Health Science Center at Brooklyn
College of Health Related Prof.
Nurse-Midwifery Program
Box 1227, 450 Clarkson Avenue
Brooklyn, NY 11203
(718) 270-7740 or 7741
Program Director:
Lily Hsia, CNM, MS

University of Medicine and Dentistry of New Jersey *94
School of Health Related Prof.
Nurse-Midwifery Program
65 Bergen Street
Newark, NJ 07107-3001
(201) 982-4249, 4298
Program Director:
Elaine Diegmann, CNM, MEd

UCSF/SFGH *94
Interdepartmental Nurse-Midwifery Education Program
(Certificate Track)
SFGH, Ward 6D, Room 24
1001 Potrero Avenue
San Francisco, CA 94110
(415) 206-5106
(Acting) Program Director:
Linda Ennis, CNM

University of Southern California *94
Nurse-Midwifery Educational Program
Women's Hospital, Room 8K5
1240 North Mission Road
Los Angeles, CA 90033
(213) 226-3386
Program Director:
Susan M. Huser, CNM, MS
(*MSN option avail. from USC-Dept. Nrsg.*)

Master's Programs

Boston University† School of Public Health
MPH/CNM Program
Room A-302
80 E. Concord Street
Boston, MA 02118
(617) 638-5042
Program Director:
Lisa Paine, CNM, DrPH, FAAN

Case Western Reserve Univ. (MSN or ND) *94
Frances Payne Bolton
School of Nursing
Nurse-Midwifery Program
10900 Euclid Avenue
Cleveland, OH 44106-4904
(216) 368-3532
Program Director:
Claire Andrews, CNM, PhD, FAAN

Columbia University (MS) *95
Graduate Program in
Nurse-Midwifery
School of Nursing
617 West 168th Street
New York, NY 10032
(212) 305-2808, 3418
Program Director:
Ronnie Lichtman, CNM, MS, M.Phil.

East Carolina University†
Nurse-Midwifery Program
School of Nursing
Greenville, NC 27858
(919) 757-6057
Program Director:
Nancy Moss, CNM, MSN, PhD

Emory University (RN/MN, MN or MN/MPH) *96
Nell Hodgson Woodruff
School of Nursing
Atlanta, GA 30322
(404) 727-6918
Program Director:
Maureen Kelley, CNM, MSN

Georgetown University (MS) *95
School of Nursing
Graduate Program in Nurse-Midwifery
3700 Reservoir Road, NW
Washington, DC 20007
(202) 687-4772
Program Director:
Deborah Bash, CNM, EdD

Medical University of South Carolina (MSN) *94
Nurse-Midwifery Program
College of Nursing
171 Ashley Avenue
Charleston, SC 29425
(803) 792-3077
Program Director:
Elizabeth M. Bear, CNM, PhD, FAAN

Oregon Health Sciences University (MS or MN) *94
School of Nursing
Dept. of Family Nursing
Nurse-Midwifery Program
3181 SW Sam Jackson Park Road
Portland, OR 97201
(503) 494-3822
Program Director:
Carol Howe, CNM, DNSc

University of Alabama School of Nursing (MSN) *98
Graduate Programs
Nurse-Midwifery Option
U of Alabama at Birmingham
UAB Station
Birmingham, AL 35294-1210
(205) 934-6648
Program Director:
Marilyn Musacchio, CNM, PhD

UCSF/SFGH (MS) *94
Interdepartmental Nurse-Midwifery Education Program
(Acting) Program Director:
Linda Ennis, CNM
UCSF School of Nursing
N411X, Box 0606
San Francisco, CA 94143-0606
(415) 476-4694
Program Co-Director:
Jeanne DeJoseph, CNM, PhD

UCSF/UCSD (MS) *94
Intercampus Graduate Studies
Dept. of Community and Family
Medicine, 0809
UCSD School of Medicine
Univ. of California, San Diego
9500 Gilman Drive
LaJolla, CA 92093-0809
(619) 543-5480
USCD Program Co-Director:
Vanda Lops, CNM, MSN

-or-

UCSF School of Nursing
N411X, Box 0606
San Francisco, CA 94143-0606
(415) 476-4694
UCSF Program Co-Director:
Jeanne DeJoseph, CNM, PhD

University of Colorado (MS) *98
Health Sciences Center
School of Nursing, Graduate Program
Nurse-Midwifery Program
4200 East 9th Avenue, Box C 288
Denver, CO 80262
(303) 270-8654
Program Director:
Deborah Perlis, CNM, PhD

University of Florida (MSN or MN) *94
Health Sciences Center, Jacksonville
Nurse-Midwifery Program
College of Nursing
653 West 8th St. Bldg 1, 2nd Floor
Jacksonville, FL 32209-6561
(904) 549-3245
Program Director:
Alice H. Poe, CNM, MN

University of Illinois at Chicago (MS) *94
College of Nursing M/C 802
Nurse-Midwifery Program
845 South Damen Avenue
Chicago, IL 60612
(312) 996-7982
Program Director:
Betty Schlatter, CNM, PhD

University of Kentucky (MSN) *94
College of Nursing
760 Rose Street
Lexington, KY 40536-0232
(606) 233-6650
Program Director:
JoAnn B. Ruiz-Bueno, CNM, PhD

University of Miami (MSN) *96
School of Nursing
D2-5, Royce Building
PO Box 016960
1755 NW 12th Avenue
Miami, FL 33136
(305) 548-4636, 4640
Program Director:
Theresa Gesse, CNM, PhD

University of Michigan *98
Nurse-Midwifery Program
School of Nursing
400 N. Ingalls, Rm. 3320
Ann Arbor, MI 48109
(313) 763-3710
Program Director:
Barbara A. Petersen, CNM, EdD

University of Minnesota (MS) *94
School of Nursing, 6-101 Unit F
308 Harvard Street SE
Minneapolis, MN 55455
(612) 624-6494
Program Director:
Mary A. Rossi, CNM, MS

University of New Mexico†
College of Nursing
Nurse-Midwifery Program
Albuquerque, NM 87131
(505) 277-1184
Program Director:
Nancy Clark, CNM, PhD

University of Pennsylvania (MSN) *94
School of Nursing
Nursing Education Building
420 Guardian Drive
Philadelphia, PA 19104-6096
(215) 898-4335
Program Director:
Joyce E. Thompson, CNM, DrPH, FAAN

University of Rhode Island†
College of Nursing
White Hall
Kingston, RI 02881-0814
(401) 792-2766
Program Director:
Diane Angelini, CNM, CNA, EdD

University of Texas at El Paso/Texas Tech University†
Collaborative Nurse-Midwifery Prog.
Texas Tech Univ. HSC
Dept of OB/GYN
4800 Alberta Avenue
El Paso, TX 79905
(915) 545-6490
Program Director:
Carolyn Routledge, CNM, MSN

University of Utah (MS) *98
 College of Nursing
 Graduate Program in Nurse-Midwifery
 25 South Medical Drive
 Salt Lake City, UT 84112
 (801) 581-8274
 Program Director:
 Diane (Dd) Fedorchak, CNM, MS

Yale University (MSN) *94
 School of Nursing
 Nurse-Midwifery Program
 25 Park Street
 PO Box 9740
 New Haven, CT 06536-0740
 (203) 737-2344
 Program Director:
 Barbara Decker, CNM, EdD

Precertification Programs

Jackson Memorial Hospital†
 University of Miami Medical Center
 Nurse-Midwifery Program
 Women's Hospital Center
 East Tower, 3003
 1611 NW 12th Avenue
 Miami, FL 33136
 (305) 585-6628
 Program Director:
 Nancy Griffis, CNM, MN-MPH

*Preaccredited status.
†Year of review for continued accreditation.
Source: ACNM.

✺ Appendix 4

Insurance Reimbursement

Many major health insurance companies and HMOs provide coverage for midwifery services. However, we can't provide a specific list of those companies because reimbursement for services depends on the individual policy of each branch of that insurance company and on state law. If an insurer refuses coverage and you don't reside in a state that requires reimbursement (see below), be sure to take it up with your employer or the insurance company. Most employers and insurance companies will comply with your request for reimbursement once they realize the cost/savings benefits of using nurse-midwife services.

As of this writing, the following states have legislation mandating private insurance reimbursement for nurse-midwifery services: Alaska, California, Colorado, Connecticut, Florida, Maryland, Massachusetts, Minnesota, Mississippi, Montana, New Hampshire, New Jersey, New Mexico, New York, Nevada, North Dakota, Ohio, Oregon, Pennsylvania, Rhode Island, South Dakota, Utah, Washington, and West Virginia.

❋ Notes

Chapter 1: Choosing a Nurse-Midwife

However, the physicians generally weren't much better off J. Whitridge Williams, "Medical Education and the Midwife Problem in the United States," *Journal of the American Medical Association,* 58, January 6, 1912, 1–7. (Page 18)

In fact, a 1918 study Grace Meigs, "Maternal Mortality from All Conditions Connected with Childbirth in the United States and Certain Other Countries," *United States Department of Labor, Children's Bureau Publication,* no. 19. Washington, DC: Government Printing Office, 1917. (Page 19)

Then, in 1925 E. Ernst and K. Gordon, "Fifty-three Years of Home Birth Experience at the Frontier Nursing Service, Kentucky, 1925–1978." In D. Stewart and L. Stewart (eds.), *Compulsory Hospitalization: Freedom of Choice in Childbirth,* Vol. 2. Marble Hill, MO: National Association of Parents & Professionals for Safe Alternatives in Childbirth, 1979. (Page 19)

The practice of midwifery in Canada Karyn J. Kaufman, "Canadian Midwifery: Attaining Recognition," *The Canadian Journal of Ob/Gyn and Women's Health Care,* 4 (4), 1992, 318–322. (Page 22)

In 1985, the Institute of Medicine Institute of Medicine, Sarah S. Brown (Ed.), *Prenatal Care: Reaching Mothers, Reaching Infants.* Washington, DC: National Academy Press, 1988. (Page 27)

In a 1986 evaluation U.S. Congress, Office of Technology Assessment, *Nurse-Practitioners, Physician Assistants, and Certified Nurse-Midwives: A Policy Analysis.* Washington, DC: Government Printing Office, 1986. (Page 27)

Chapter 2: Can I Go to a Midwife?

Studies conducted in diverse areas Marie Meglen, "A Prototype of Health Services for Quality of Life in a Rural County," *Bulletin of Nurse-Midwifery,* 17(4), November 1972, 103–13; Sister Angela Murdaugh, "Experiences of a New Migrant Health Clinic," *Women and Health,* 1(6), November–December 1976, 25–28; and M. Brenda Doyle and Mary V. Widhalm, "Midwifing the Adolsecents at Lincoln Hospital's Teen-Age Clinics," *Journal of Nurse-Midwifery,* 24(4), July-August 1979, 27–32. (Page 30)

In fact, nurse-midwives were praised by U.S. Congress, Office of Technology Assessment, *Nurse Practitioners, Physician Assistants and Certified Nurse-Midwives: A Policy Analysis.* Washington, DC: Government Printing Office, 1986. (Page 34)

Numerous studies have shown (Is a midwife safe) Southern Regional Task Force on Infant Mortality, Interim Report, Southern Governors' Association, February 24, 1985. (Page 37)

As a result, several prominent organizations Sara Rosenbaums, *The Children's Defense Fund Adolescent Pregnancy*

Prevention/Prenatal Care Campaign. Washington, DC, 1985. (Page 38)

Chapter 4: Your Birth Experience

A 1989 study James Thorp et al., "The Effect of Continuous Epidural Analgesia on Cesarean Section for Dystocia in Nulliparous Women," *American Journal of Obstetrics and Gynecology, 161*(3), 1989, 670–675. (Page 72)

Studies confirm that staying mobile Roberto Caldeyro-Barcia, "Supine Called the Worst Position for Labor and Delivery," *Family Practice News,* 5(11), 1975. (Page 73)

Chapter 7: Birth Centers

According to Kitty Ernst E. Ernst, Editorial, "'Health Care for All'" by the year 2000," *NACC News,* 50(1), 1990. (Page 101)

In the National Birth Center study Judith Rooks, CNM, M.S., MPH; Norman Weatherby, Ph.D.; Eunice K. M. Ernst, CNM, MPH; et al., "Outcomes of Care in Birth Centers," National Birth Center Study, *New England Journal of Medicine,* December 28, 1989, pp. 1804–1825. (Page 108)

A recent study by the American Hospital Association American Hospital Association, 1990 Study, as reported in the *Philadelphia Inquirer,* June 13, 1991, p. 13. (Page 111)

Chapter 8: Home Birth

A 1984 study of home birth outcomes Rona Campbell et al., "Home Births in England and Wales: Perinatal Mortality According to Intended Place of Delivery," *British Medical Journal* 289, 1984, 721–724. (Page 121)

The most comprehensive study Lewis Mehl et al., "Outcomes of Elective Home Births," *Journal of Reproductive Medicine,* November 1977, pp. 281–290; revised in 1980. (Page 121)

Chapter 9: Not Just Birth

A 1993 study "Survey Finds Health Care Gap for Women," *San Jose Mercury News,* July 15, 1993. (Page 130)

Chapter 10: Minding Your Body

The mind/body interaction is an actual physical process From the PBS series Healing and the Mind. (Page 142)

In her book Lucy Waletsky, M.D., *Psychologic Benefits of Nurse-Midwifery Care.* In ACNM, *Nurse-Midwifery in America,* 1986. (Page 146)

Chapter 11: The Future of Certified Nurse-Midwives

A 1993 meta-analysis Sharon A. Brown, Ph.D., R.N., Associate Professor of Nursing and Associate Dean for Research, University of Texas–Houston Health Science Center School of Nursing; and Deanna E. Grimes, Dr.Ph., R.N., Associate Professor of Nursing, University of Texas–Houston Health Center School of Nursing, *A Meta-Analysis of Process of Care, Clinical Outcomes, and Cost Effectiveness of Nurses in Primary Care Roles: Nurse Practitioners and Nurse Midwives.* American Nurses Association, January 1993. (Page 158)

According to Ruth Lubic Laura Clark, "How Fast Are Patients Abandoning Doctors for Midwives?" *Medical Economics Magazine,* November 1990, p. 10. (Page 164)

✖ Glossary

Alpha fetoprotein: Substance produced by the fetus that is measured in the mother's blood to screen for increased risk for certain problems in the baby such as spina bifida or Down syndrome.

Amniocentesis: Withdrawing some amniotic fluid from the amniotic sac by inserting a needle through the abdomen. The fluid is studied for a number of possible genetic disorders among babies.

Amniotic Sac: Sac containing amniotic fluid in which the baby floats; also called bag of waters.

Amniotomy: Rupturing the amniotic sac with an instrument.

Anesthetic/Anesthesia: Medication injected along a nerve pathway to deaden pain. Can be general, in which you are put to sleep; regional, in which a region of your body is put to sleep, as with a spinal or epidural; or local, in which a small part of your body is numbed.

Apgar Score: An evaluation of a newborn's adjustment to life outside the womb, performed at 1 and 5 minutes.

Bag of Waters: See **Amniotic Sac**.

Birth Canal: The area between the uterus and outside of the body which the baby passes through; also called the vagina.

Bonding: Forming a relationship with a baby through general interaction, holding, touching, and so on.

Breech: A baby positioned bottom down instead of head down in the uterus.

Cervix: The necklike part of the uterus that opens into the birth canal.

Cesarean Birth (C-Section): Birth of a baby by cutting through the abdomen into the uterus and lifting the baby out.

Chorionic Villus Sampling (CVS): Genetic screening test that takes a sample of early fetal cells using a thin catheter inserted into the uterus either through the vagina or abdominal wall.

Circumcision: Removal of the foreskin of the penis of a baby.

Contraction: Also called labor pain; tightening of the uterine muscle that dilates the cervix during labor.

Demand Feeding: Feeding the baby whenever he or she is hungry.

Dilation: Opening of the cervix by contractions in labor, measured by centimeters. At 10 centimeters (full dilation) you are ready to push the baby out.

Doppler: Ultrasound device for listening to the fetal heartbeat.

Electronic Fetal Monitor: Machine that continuously keeps track of the baby's heartbeat and the mother's contractions during labor; attached internally to the baby's head or externally on the mother's abdomen.

Epidural: Also called regional anesthesia. Injection of medication into the epidural space of the spine to numb the lower half of the body.

Episiotomy: Surgical enlargement of the vagina during delivery of a baby.

Fetal Distress: A condition in which the baby is deprived of oxygen. Can be seen by changes in the pattern of the baby's heartbeat.

Fetoscope: Special stethoscope used to listen to the baby's heartbeat during pregnancy and labor.

Forceps: Metal instruments that fit around the baby's head to help pull the baby out during delivery.

General Anesthetic: See **Anesthesia**.

High Risk: Having a medical condition like diabetes or high blood pressure that requires special care during pregnancy and birth.

Hormone: A chemical messenger in the blood that stimulates various organs to action.

Induction of Labor: Artificially caused labor to start by rupturing the bags of water or giving pitocin or prostaglandin or other drugs.

Intravenous (IV): Infusion of fluids, such as glucose, through a thin tube into a vein in the arm.

Labor: The process that results in the birth of a baby, comprised of three stages: (1) dilation of the cervix, (2) pushing the baby out, and (3) delivery of the placenta.

Meconium: The first bowel movement of the baby, usually passed after birth. When it is passed before birth it stains the amniotic fluid and is possibly a sign of distress; is referred to as meconium staining.

Neonatology: Branch of medicine that specializes in the high-risk newborn.

Obstetrician/Gynecologist: Physician who specializes in women's reproductive health.

Oxytocin: Naturally occurring hormone that stimulates labor.

Perinatal: The period of time before, during, and after birth.

Perinatologist: Obstetrician who specializes in high-risk pregnancies.

Perineum: The area between the rectum and vaginal opening. It is the perineum that is cut in an episiotomy.

Pitocin: Synthetic hormone that acts like the hormone oxytocin, stimulating contractions. Also used to help control postpartum bleeding.

Placenta: The organ that nourishes the fetus during pregnancy. It is attached to the mother's uterus and to the baby by the umbilical cord.

Rooming-in: Having your baby stay in your room in the hospital instead of in the nursery.

Transition: The period of labor usually prior to pushing.

Ultrasound: A procedure where sound waves are bounced off an object such as a fetus to create a picture on a television-like screen.

Uterus: Organ where the baby grows during pregnancy.

Vacuum: An instrument that suctions on to the baby's head in order to pull her or him out of the vagina. Used as an alternative to forceps in some cases.

Vagina: See **Birth Canal**.

✳ Index

Abdominal pain, 54
Abruptio placenta, 54
Alcohol abuse, 32
Alpha fetoprotein test (AFP), 50
American College of Nurse-Midwives
    (ACNM), 16, 17, 20, 21, 22, 159,
    160, 164
American College of Nurse-Midwives
    Foundation, 146, 157
American College of Obstetricians and
    Gynecologists, 16, 69, 159, 163
American Hospital Association, 111
*American Journal of Obstetrics and
    Gynecology,* 72
American Journal of Public Health, 17
American Medical Association, 161
American Nurses Association, 158
Amniocentesis, 45, 51, 66
Anemia, 36
Anesthesia, 23, 38, 66, 72, 87, 98

Backache, 50
Back labor, 79
Bassett (Imogene) Hospital,
    Cooperstown, NY, 94–95
Battered woman syndrome, 135, 136
Bay Area Midwives, 120
Birth as an American Rite of Passage
    (Davis-Floyd), 85
Birth centers, 87, 101–113
    accreditation of, 102, 112
    birthing experience at, 7–8, 104–105
    client screening, 104, 106, 108
    cost of, 107, 110–111, 118
    examples of, 106–108
    and health-care reform, 164
    history of, 103–104
    information sources, 176
    nature of, 101–103
    safety of, 4–5, 108–110
    selection criteria, 111–113

Birthing room, 98
Birth Place, The, Menlo Park,
    California, 106–107, 110–111
Birth plan, 65–67
Bleeding, vaginal, 47–48, 54
Blood pressure, 48, 60, 69
Blood tests, 44, 50–51
"Bloody show," 68
Bonding process, 82
Boston Women's Health Book
    Collective, 103
Braxton-Hicks contractions, 58–59
Brazelton, T. Berry, 82, 94, 162
Breaking the water, 54
Breast-feeding, 56, 98, 174–175
Breckenridge, Mary, 19
Breech births, vaginal, 35
Brigham and Women's Hospital,
    Boston, 93–94
Brody, Jane, 27, 108–109, 166
Burst, Helen, 158

Calcium carbonate, 50
Canada, midwifery in, 21–22
Carnegie Foundation for the
    Advancement of Teaching, 158
Carr, Catherine, 163
Castor oil, 60
Center for Disease Control, 161
Certification exam, 21
Certified Nurse-Midwife (CNM). See
    Nurse-midwife.
Cervical mucus, 131
Cesarean section, 29, 35, 38, 66, 79,
    80, 122
    epidurals and, 72
    previous, 30, 104, 106
    rate, 76, 94, 95, 96, 97, 161
    unnecessary, 161
    vaginal birth after (VBAC), 120, 148
Childbearing Center, New York, 103
Childbirth education class, 55–56
Childbirth. See Labor and birth.
Children's Defense Fund, 38
Chorionic villus sampling (CVS), 45

Circumcision, 56–57
Clinton, Bill, 163
Colorectal cancer screen, 135
Colposcopy, 23
Commission for the Accreditation of
    Childbearing Centers, 102, 112
Commonwealth Fund, 18, 130
Community-Based Nurse-Midwifery
    Education Program, 164–165
Complications
    at birth centers, 109–110
    breech birth, 35
    of first trimester, 47–48
    in labor, 79–80
    of second trimester, 53–54
    of third trimester, 59–60
    twins, 34–35
Cramping, 54
Creevy, Don, 27–28, 162, 163–164

Daniel, Joyce, 118–119
Davis-Floyd, Robbie, 85, 86,
    161–162
Demerol, 64
Diabetes, 30, 32, 48, 135
    gestational, 51
Diet and nutrition, 46, 50
Dilation, 55
Dilation and evacuation (D & E), 48
Direct-entry midwife, 25
Dohrn, Jennifer, 116
Doppler, 69
Doula, 65, 76, 123, 173
Down syndrome, 51
Drug abuse, 32
Due date, 60

Effacement, 55
Elsberry, Charlotte Pixie, 95
Emergency childbirth procedures, 61
Emergency equipment, 4, 112, 124
Endorphins, 142
Epidural anesthesia, 30, 72, 87
Episiotomy, 23, 38, 59, 64, 66, 77–78
Ernst, Kitty, 164

Exercise and pregnancy, 46, 51, 59
Eyedrops, for newborn, 57, 81

False labor, 59
Family Birth Associates, 118–119
Family planning, 133–134
Family support, 33, 52–53, 75–76
Federal Trade Commission, 160
Fetal distress, 80, 110
Fetal monitor, 5, 23, 30, 60, 66, 69
Fetoscope, 69
Forceps delivery, 38, 66, 72, 79, 98
Frontier Nursing Service, 19–20,
    164–165
Fundal height, 48

General Accounting Office, 38
Genetic testing, 24, 30, 45
Gestational diabetes, 51
Grubb, Shelly, 7, 12

Haas, J., 146
Healing and the Mind (Moyers), 142
Health-care reform, 160–164
Health insurance, 99, 110, 111, 116,
    119, 159, 189
Health Letter, 161
Health maintenance organizations
    (HMOs), 20, 71, 110, 119, 189
Healthy Start Program, 162
Heartburn, 50
Heart disease, 31
Heller, Mark, 94
High-risk pregnancy, 30, 31–32, 150,
    162
Holy Family Services Birth Center,
    Weslaco, Texas, 107
Home birth, 86, 87, 115–125
    advantages of, 117–118
    barriers to, 116–117
    cost of, 118–119
    decline in, 115–116, 125
    examples of, 119–121
    information sources, 177
    preparing for, 123

safety of, 121–122
selection criteria, 122–125
Hormone replacement therapy,
    138–139
Hospital birth, 86, 87, 89–98
    cost of, 99, 111, 118
    hospital selection, 91–95, 96–99
    pros and cons of, 89–91
    safety of, 95–96
    transfers, 109–110, 112, 120, 123–124
Hospital privileges, 158
Howse, Jennifer, 160, 161
Hypertension, 31
    pregnancy-induced, 60

Induced labor, 60, 79–80
Infant mortality, 19, 35, 122, 161
Infertility, 37, 42
Insurance reimbursement, 186
Institute of Medicine, 27, 38
Intrauterine device (IUD), 133
IVs, 73, 80, 104, 112

Jennings, Richard, 145
Jewish General Hospital, 77–78
Johns Hopkins School of Public
    Health, 150
Jones, Rhoda Dankin, 97
*Journal of the American Medical
    Association*, 76
Journal of Nurse Midwifery, 163
Journal of Reproductive Medicine, 121

Kaiser Permanente, 119
Kaufman, Karyn, 22
Kegel exercise, 51
Kennell, John, 76
Kidney disease, 31
Klaus, Marshall, 76
Klaus, Phyliss, 76

Labor and birth, 63–82
    active, 69–74
    birth plan, 65–67
    bonding with newborn, 82

Labor and birth, (continued)
    comfort measures in, 69–71
    companions in, 65, 75–76, 147–148
    complications in, 35, 79–80
    difficult, 78–79
    early, 67–68
    emergency procedures, 61
    episiotomy in, 23, 38, 59, 64, 66,
        77–78
    fears about, 63–64
    induced, 60, 79–80
    information sources, 169
    medical technology in, 77
    midwife on call for, 49, 148
    mind-body connection, 145–149,
        151–152
    newborn examination, 80–81
    pain relief in, 71–72
    position in, 73–74
    preparation for, 54–56, 58–59
    pushing, 74–75
    slow progress, 34, 146–147
Labor room, 97–98
Laing, Karen, 116, 118
Lay midwife, 25
Licensing requirements, 21
Lobenstine Midwifery School, 20
Lubic, Ruth, 164

McGill University, 77–78
Malpractice insurance, 120, 125,
    159–160
Mammogram, 135
Maternal mortality, 19
Maternity Center Association, 103
Medical technology, 77, 85, 91
Medical University of South Carolina, 35
Mehl, Lewis, 121–122
Membranes, premature rupture of, 54
Menopause, 137–139
Menstrual cramps, 134
Menstrual cycles, irregular, 134,
    150–151
Mental health, 135
    See also Mind/body connection.

Midwife
    types of, 25, 158
    See also Nurse-midwife.
Midwives Alliance of North America
    (MANA), 25
Mind/body connection, 141–153
    information sources, 172
    in labor and birth, 145–149,
        151–152
    midwife approach to, 142–143
    nature of, 141–142
    postpartum, 149–150
    in pregnancy, 144–145, 151
    in well-woman care, 150–151
Miscarriage
    previous, 30
    surgical procedure in, 48
Mothering the Mother (Kennell, Klaus,
    and Klaus), 76
Moyers, Bill, 142
Murdaugh, Angela, 107

National Association of Childbearing
    Centers, 104
National Birth Center Study, 108, 109
National Institute of Child Health and
    Human Development, 45
Neonatologist, 37
Newborn
    bonding with, 82
    breast-feeding, 56, 98, 174–175
    circumcision, 56–58
    nursery, 97
    screening tests, 8, 57, 81
New England Journal of Medicine,
    108
New York Academy of Medicine, 18
North Central Bronx Hospital, New
    York, 95
Nurse-midwife
    barriers to profession, 157–158
    birthplace settings, 20, 86–87. See
        also Birth centers; Home birth;
        Hospital birth.
    in Canada, 21–22

client screening, 30–34, 42–44, 104, 106, 108
defined, 17, 22
earnings, 163
education programs for, 11, 21, 22, 34, 165, 179–188
and health-care reform, 160–164
and high-risk pregnancy, 30, 31–32, 162
historical background, 17–20, 170
holistic approach of, 16, 142–143
information sources, 171
malpractice insurance for, 159–160
organizations, 173–174
philosophy of care, 24, 152
and physicians, 15–16, 43, 145–146
physician backup, 4, 23, 26, 35–37, 47
reasons for choosing, 2–3, 26–28
recruitment of, 164–165
as routine caregiver, 165–166
safety record of, 37–38, 159
scope of practice, 22–23
selection criteria, 25–26
See also Labor and birth; Prenatal care; Well-woman care.
Nurse-Midwifery in America, 146

Obstetrician/gynecologist, 4, 15, 37, 145–146, 162
Office of Technology Assessment, 27, 34, 38
Ontario, Canada, 22
Organization for Economic Development and Cooperation, 161
Our Bodies Ourselves, 103
Ovarian cysts, 134
Overweight, 46
Oxytocin, 80

Pain medication, 71–72, 105, 106
Palmer, Harriet, 118, 119, 120
Papaya enzyme, 50
Pap smear, 3, 23, 36, 44, 130, 133, 135

Parent education classes, 55–56
Parr, Elizabeth A., 1, 10–12, 24, 31, 33, 35, 55, 64, 70, 73, 74–75, 96, 105, 131, 132, 133–134, 135, 138–139, 148–149, 152
Pediatrician, 4, 37, 57–58
Peer review, 21
Pelvic exam, 55, 132, 137
Pelvic rocking, 51
Perinatologist, 37
Perineal massage, 59, 75
Pert, Candace, 142
Phenylketonuria, 57
Physical exam
    prenatal care, 3, 44
    well-woman care, 130–133
Physician
    consulting, 4, 23, 26, 35–37, 47
    earnings, 163
    future role of, 162
    and nurse-midwives, 15–16, 43, 145–146
    pediatrician selection, 57–58
Pitocin, 6, 66, 80, 98, 110
PKU test, 8, 57
Placenta problems, 54
Poole, Catherine M., 1, 2–10, 24, 27, 55–56, 61, 75, 102, 105, 130, 133–134, 153
Postpartum depression, 149–150
Pre-eclampsia, 60
Premature baby rate, 158
Premenstrual syndrome (PMS), 134
Prenatal care, 3–4, 41–61
    baby care advice, 56–58
    childbirth preparation, 54–56, 58–59, 64
    client involvement, 5, 49
    complications, 34–35, 47–48, 53–54, 59–60
    diet, 46–47, 50, 51
    exercise, 46, 51, 59
    family support in, 33, 52–53
    first trimester, 42–48
    information sources, 171

Prenatal care *(continued)*
  mind/body connection, 144–145, 151
  physical exam, 3, 44, 48, 55
  of pregnancy discomforts, 50
  pregnancy education, 51–52
  screening client, 30–34, 42–44
  second trimester, 48–54
  sexual concerns in, 53
  tests and procedures, 44–46, 50–51
  third trimester, 54–61
Prescription-writing privileges, 159
Preterm labor, 34, 54
Previa, 54
Prostaglandin, 79
Public Citizen Health Research Group,
  97, 161
Pushing stage of labor, 74–75, 141

Reading Birth and Women's Center,
  Pennsylvania, 110
Registered nurse (R.N.), 7
Regulated Health Professions Act of
  1991, 22
Relaxation techniques, 69–70
Resuscitation, 23, 34
Rooks, J., 146
Rooming-in, 98

St. James, Susan, 20
Sexual counseling, 53, 136–137, 151
Shephard, Cybil, 20
Slow progress labor, 34, 146–147
Sonogram. *See* Ultrasound.
Spina bifida, 51
Squatting exercise, 59
Stanford University Hospital, 106
Stress test, 5–6, 60
Su Clinica, 107
Swelling, abnormal, 60

Task Force on Health Care, 163
Technology, medical, 77, 85, 91
Teenagers, in well-woman care,
  132–133, 137

Third party reimbursement, 159
Thompson, Joyce, 163
Thyroid screening, 57
Toxemia, 48
Twin births, 34–35, 36

Ultrasound, 30, 45–46, 51, 60
Urinary tract infections, 134–135
Urine test, 44, 48, 49
"Uterine ear" theory, 145

Vacuum extractor, 23, 72
Vaginal births after Cesarean section
  (VBACs), 120, 148
Vaginal infections, 134
Varicose veins, 50
Vasectomy, 133–134
Vitamin K, 57, 81

Waletsky, Lucy, 146
Warning signs, 47–48
Well-woman care, 3, 23, 36, 129–138
  annual checkup, 130–133
  family planning, 133–134
  gynecological problems, 134–135
  health screening/prevention,
    135–136
  information sources, 170, 175–176
  menopause, 137–139
  mind/body connection, 150–151
  nature of, 129–130
  sexual counseling, 136–137
White House Conference on Child
  Health and Protection of Fetal
  Newborn and Material Morbidity
  and Mortality, 18
Williams, J. Whitridge, 18
Wolfe, Sidney, 97
Women's Health Alert, Massachusetts,
  96–97

Yale University Child Study Center,
  150
Yeast infection, 135